Decentralizing Health Services

Krishna Regmi
Editor

Decentralizing Health Services

A Global Perspective

Foreword by Prof. David J. Hunter

Springer

Editor
Krishna Regmi
Department of Clinical Education
and Leadership
Faculty of Health & Social Sciences
University of Bedfordshire
UK

ISBN 978-1-4614-9070-8 ISBN 978-1-4614-9071-5 (eBook)
DOI 10.1007/978-1-4614-9071-5
Springer New York Heidelberg Dordrecht London

Library of Congress Control Number: 2013954799

Printed on acid-free paper

Springer is part of Springer Science+Business Media (www.springer.com)

Foreword

Health systems globally are once again going through a period of considerable turbulence. The reasons are many and complex. Some have their roots in the economic crisis triggered by the collapse of the financial sector in 2008 which heralded a period of austerity in many countries. Others arise from the demographic changes evident arising from an ageing population which require that health systems change and give higher priority to primary health care and social care than to hospital services. And yet other reasons arise from the nature of the wicked problems that confront contemporary health systems to which there is no simple or single solution—problems arising from lifestyle-related non-communicable diseases that have more to do with public health—and which require new forms of governance including engagement from multiple levels of government in order to tackle them. Also evident as part of the tsunami of reform sweeping through many countries is a particular focus on choice, competition and markets as instruments to improve the performance of services. The reasons for their appeal are not altogether clear when the evidence base for them remains so weak and contested. It is hard to conclude other than that such actions possibly have more to do with the prevailing political ideology than the state of the evidence base. Politics is therefore to the fore in keeping with the eighteenth-century Prussian pathologist turned anthropologist turned parliamentarian, Rudolf Virchow, who famously remarked that 'medicine is a social science, and politics nothing else but medicine on a large scale'.

As the contributors to this important and timely book testify, decentralization is typically a central plank of health sector reform. It is seen as an effective means to stimulate improvements in the delivery of services, to secure better allocation of resources according to needs, to involve the community in decisions about priorities and to facilitate the reduction of inequities in health. Whether the ambitious claims for decentralization outweigh the disadvantages, notably fragmented and duplicated services as well as high transaction costs, are not known, but they demand careful scrutiny especially when the emphasis in health policy in many countries is on securing better joined-up services, notably health and social care, in order to meet the needs of those who do not require expensive hospital care but rather integrated services to enable them to lead independent lives and remain living at home or in the community.

This book sets out to explore such considerations and tensions. As the chapters demonstrate, decentralization, while often seen as a panacea to the myriad flaws evident in health-care systems, can bring with it undesirable and unintended side effects. Moreover, governments are often ambivalent in their preferences which can prove short lived. Some, while proclaiming the virtues of decentralization, or localism in the English NHS parlance, invariably revert to a default position with its emphasis on centralisation and top-down control. And where health systems are funded through central taxation, it is indeed difficult for governments to let go and effectively devolve responsibility when accountability inevitably and unavoidably remains a matter for national legislative assemblies. But context is all important in such matters and what works (or not) in one country may not elsewhere. Learning from different countries' experiences has therefore to be undertaken with considerable care and caution since there are limits to what can be transposed from one system to another and with what effect.

The cyclical, and often paradoxical, nature of health system reform is evident in many of the contributions to the book. Governments become disappointed and disenchanted with centralised services that are perceived to be slow to innovate and are unresponsive to patient and public preferences. Invariably national ministries of health are required to tackle such concerns and then are blamed for a failure to do so when the results are disappointing or fail to materialise. Decentralization therefore becomes attractive as a way of distancing such concerns from central government—if nothing else, blame can be diffused. At the same time, governments can confidently assert that they are letting go and liberating services in order that they can be organised and prioritised locally and remain sensitive to local wishes and preferences. Decentralization can be seductive in such circumstances. And yet, once having let go, and often for the best of intentions, the self-same governments, or their immediate successors, then quickly find that they lack the means or levers to deal with issues of varying standards, growing inequity and an inability to influence the direction of health care. Even if governments maintain some influence over strategy and the direction of health policy, many find it difficult to avoid influencing not just what it is that health services do but how they go about doing it. And so the cycle begins again. Health policy becomes a swinging pendulum between the poles of centralisation and decentralization, respectively. Many countries, notably the UK, but especially England since political devolution in 1999, have oscillated between an emphasis on centralisation and top-down control of health policy on the one hand and decentralization and allowing the periphery a greater degree of freedom to decide its own priorities on the other hand. Finding an optimal balance between the two extremes has eluded governments both in the UK and in many other countries.

Part of the problem lies in the different skill set required by central government in order to allow decentralization to develop and prosper. Once services are no longer directly run by the centre, its role of necessity has to move to one concerned with monitoring, regulation and inspection. But generally, bodies charged with regulation and inspection in many health systems are weak and lack effective levers. It is also important to get the balance right between overregulation on the one hand, which risks driving out creativity and diversity, and under-regulation on the other hand, which unwittingly allows service providers to deliver substandard services which in extreme cases could put lives at risk. Finding the optimal balance between these extremes has proved difficult and defeated many governments which have tried.

It is not the subject of the book although it comes to the fore, or surfaces, in most of the chapters, but a key feature, or outcome, of decentralization is a greater reliance on the private sector and markets for the provision of health services. In fact, decentralization and privatisation are conceptually distinct processes which may or may not be interrelated. Yet why governments of various political persuasions choose to outsource services to the private sector when the evidence base to underpin such decisions is either lacking or hotly contested can only seemingly be explained by ideology and in particular by neo-liberalism which is in the ascendancy in the majority of countries despite the events in the global financial sector in 2008 which had its roots in poor regulation.

Another feature of the centralisation versus decentralization discourse is the place of health inequalities and how these might best be tackled. Given that they are growing to a greater or lesser degree in virtually all health systems as the work of Michael Marmot has shown, the issue is whether decentralization serves to widen the health gap between social groups or whether it offers the potential for resolving such inequalities.

Decentralization can bring benefits as well as difficulties although their precise mix will vary between countries and over time. These, and other, aspects of decentralization and health system reform are reviewed in the contributions to this book. A principal theme running through the book is the need to be clear about which functions should be decentralized and which should remain under central control. Often there is vagueness about such matters which can cause confusion and breed disappointment in the outcome.

Possibly the most critical question to ask of decentralization is what its purpose is. Decentralization is a means to an end and not an end in itself. The key issue to consider is therefore not whether to employ it as an instrument of policy but how and to what effect in order to ensure that the objectives of health policy are most effectively achieved. But, when all is said and done, of one thing we can be confident—this book will not be the last word on the subject as governments continue to struggle and search for workable and lasting solutions to the dilemma of how best to provide health and health care in increasingly complex societies. Sadly, health policymakers appear in general to lack a corporate memory or an ability to learn from previous policy initiatives. It is therefore to be hoped that at the very least the contents of this book will help sharpen the arguments and avoid a repetition of some past mistakes.

Durham, UK David J. Hunter

About the Editor

Dr. Krishna Regmi, PhD, MPH, PGDipHE, has been a Principal Lecturer in Public Health and Academic Public Health Portfolio Lead at the University of Bedfordshire, UK. He has got more than 20 years of experience of public health and health system teaching and research at the national and international levels. He is the author of several book/book chapters and a number of journal articles. Krishna is a Fellow of the Royal Society of Public Health, Fellow of the Royal Society of Medicine and Senior Fellow of the Higher Education Academy, UK.

Acknowledgements

Dedicated to those health-care professionals who truly believe that reforming health services is the single most important movement in bringing lasting change in poor people's health status globally.

Khristine Queja, Christina Tuballes and Anne Meagher from Springer US, and Bharath Krishnamoorthy from SPi Technologies looked after this book as it moved through publication. I thank them for their careful work.

Contents

Contributors

Matthew Almond University of East London, London, UK

Thomas J. Bossert Harvard School of Public Health, Boston, MA, USA

Mario S. de Leon Centre for the Study of Conflict, Power and Violence (CEDESCPV) in Europe, London, UK

Norman Flynn SOAS/University of London, London, UK

Dolores Jiménez-Rubio University of Granada, Granada, Spain

Beatriz Londoño University of Antioquia, Medellin, Colombia

Ritu Mahendru Ministry of Rural Rehabilitation and Development, Kabul, Afghanistan

Gloria Molina University of Antioquia, Medellin, Colombia

Oliver Mudyarabikwa University of East London, London, UK

Krishna Regmi University of Bedfordshire, Luton, UK

Colin Thunhurst University of Coventry, Coventry, UK

Patrick Tobi Institute for Health and Human Development, University of East London, London, UK

Julian Vargas University of Antioquia, Medellin, Colombia

Chapter 1
Health Service Decentralization: An Overview

Krishna Regmi

Abstract Health services worldwide are facing serious challenges, not only because they are not responsive to address people's health-care needs but also because they have consistently failed to accommodate the central and local dynamics of wider health determinants within the changing sociopolitical, environmental and organisational context of governance and public services. Restructuring in health care is, therefore, envisaged to make health services more equitable, inclusive and fair. This chapter provides an understanding of the general concepts of decentralization – a form of reform mechanism which operates by transferring central authorities and responsibilities along with appropriate resources to local authorities, regions or sub-national bodies, with the anticipation that local authorities are 'champions' in assessing, identifying and seeking appropriate solutions for local people's problems. This also explores the nature, the challenges and the opportunities of decentralization. Many countries are taking the decentralization route in an effort to achieve effectiveness and equity of services. But is that often the case? To what extent does the pertinent evidence match with these notions? This chapter will help your understanding better through discussing these questions in the contextual paradigms.

After Reading This Chapter, You Will Be Able to

- *Understand the concept of decentralization and decentralization in health services.*
- *Explore the nature and typology of decentralization.*
- *Examine some opportunities and challenging aspects of decentralization.*

K. Regmi (✉)
Department of Clinical Education and Leadership, Faculty of Health & Social Sciences - Institute for Health Research, University of Bedfordshire, Putteridge Bury Campus, Room 32, Luton LU2 8LE, UK
e-mail: krishna.regmi@beds.ac.uk

K. Regmi (ed.), *Decentralizing Health Services: A Global Perspective*,
DOI 10.1007/978-1-4614-9071-5_1,

Introduction

Currently, health systems worldwide are facing a serious challenge, not only because they have not addressed the people's health-care needs and demands appropriately but also because the systems have consistently failed to accommodate wider health-care determinants and principles of universality, equality, opportunity and responsibility in health and well-being (WHO 2004; National School of Government 2007). Health sectors are complex structured relationships between the people and the institutions, where institutions will offer an organised social response to the people's need (Londono and Frenk 1997). Since the 1990s, decentralization, a form of reform mechanism, has *been initiated in* many transitional nations (Dzakula 2005). This is a process of transfer or dispersal of central authority and power to local authorities or sub-national bodies in making public services more responsive to meeting people's needs (Saltman and Figueras 1997; Saltman et al. 2007). The World Bank report highlights that 'out of 75 developing and transitional countries with populations greater than 5 million, all but 12 claim to be embarked on some form of transfer of political power to local units of government' (Dillinger 1994, p.8). It is therefore a general consensus that reforming of public services in the form of new models of health delivery is inevitable in response 'to a variety of economic and political pressures as well as to the population's longstanding health-care problems' through delivering more inclusive and equitable services (Figueras et al. 2005; World Bank 1993; World Bank 2004; WHO 2008a).

Why Decentralization

Decentralization concerns how government should be structured and where power, authority and responsibilities should be located (SOAS 2009). This involves bringing 'local governments closer to the people to be able to address local needs appropriately' (Smith 1985, pp. 8–9; Work 2002, p. 4). Hadenius (2003) argues that when decentralization brings government closer to people, this would enable the local community to 'participate and exert influence' as the reason given was that 'when power is brought closer to citizens, the political process becomes more tangible and transparent and more people can become involved' (p. 1).

There are several justifications given for transferring or devolving central authorities and responsibilities to local authorities, but one promising reason was to make public services more responsive towards people's needs through correcting central government's top-down 'bureaucratic' mentality (Bienen et al. 1990). This will also develop some degree of efficient and harmonious relationship between the central and local authorities (UNDP 1999). In the light of these notions, Hutton (cited in National School of Government 2007) argues that we need to develop a model of delivery which 'fundamentally rejects the old model of top-down monolithic public services, run from the centre, in favour of greater devolution, diversity and choice; that shifts the focus into meeting the individual needs of those who use these services, and onto the quality and not just the quantity of public service provision' (p. 12).

In a similar vein, WHO (2007) notes that reform should be an essential step for undertaking changes in health performance.

> 'A directed change approach from the centre need to be rejected in decentralised health system instead needs a wider decision space at the locality. A wide choices of economic and non-economic incentives scheme, both for individual and institutional, need to be tested and established to rectify current issues of human resources retention at the local level' (WHO 2007, p.2).

Another important reason to advocate decentralising health systems is that many health services are rated as being of poor quality and they are delivered by poorly motivated staff and outdated clinical practices, and as a result, the current health-care services have not been appropriately responsive to address the people's health-care needs (Figueras et al. 2004). In Cassels' (1995) view, reforms should relate to defining and refining service priorities and reforming institutions which formulate and then implement appropriate policies in the light of these priorities in practice. Collins (1996) views decentralization as a mechanism or approach to reform the institutional paradigm. Traditionally the concept of decentralization has emerged from the field of public administration focusing on how a state or national political structure operates in terms of distributing its authorities, responsibilities and accountabilities (Bossert 1996). The notion of decentralization in the health sector has not been well researched, and even the available literature has failed to link decentralization and health at appropriate levels.

Decentralization is a sociopolitical process of moving or redistributing central authorities and responsibilities to the local or peripheral governments, with some level of negotiation, in the hope that locals are 'champions' to assess and address local people's interests and needs (Mills et al. 1990; Regmi et al. 2009). In this respect, decentralization is a mechanism in health system reform – but clearly one of many forms linking to political devolution, administrative changes, increased autonomy for practitioners and local systems (Peckham et al. 2005; 2008). There are various models and approaches to employ in public sector—including health service—reform, but which to use, if any, and how such model(s) would work in practice are other challenges (National School of Government 2007). This will have different relevance in different systems (e.g. centrally funded and controlled within a strong democratic framework (UK), federal systems (Spain, Canada, USA), provincial, countries with weak institutional structures). The UK government approach to the reform of public services, for example, is directed at:

> 'Citizen-centred and response; universal, accessible to all (in the case of core services like health and education) free at the point of use; efficient and effective, offering value for money to the taxpayer; equitable, helping to reduce social exclusion and improve the life chances of the disadvantaged; excellent quality; and empowering and involving citizens in shaping public policies' (National School of Government 2007, p. 12).

Motives for Decentralization

In Latin America—it has been considered as an essential process of democratisation by installing elected governments over central autocratic regimes.

In Africa—the advent of multiparty political systems can make public services responsive to the needs of people while at the same time empowering local people in planning and decision-making.

Ethiopia—as a response to minimising inequalities and ethnic disparities, groups thereby provide opportunities to participate in the political process.

Mozambique and Uganda—an attempt to keep the country together as an outcome of long civil wars—'asymmetrical federations'.

Former socialist states (e.g. the Czech Republic, Baltic states and Poland)—to collapse old central autocratic-hierarchical regimes.

Russia, Bosnia—to minimise some ethnic tensions.

Eastern Europe and former Soviet Union—transition from a command to a market economy.

East Asia—to improve planning and delivery of public services on a larger scale.

South Asia—to overcome challenges of ethnic and geographical disparities.

In many nations across the world—decentralization acts as a *means* to providing public services through establishing good governance systems, often cross-cutting themes of the broader processes of political and economic reform—political development, institutional capacity, corruption, governance, equity and poverty reduction.

Source: Litvack et al. (1998), World Bank (1997), World Bank (n.d.).

Decentralization in Health

Decentralization policies in the health sector have been gaining popularity in most developed and developing nations since 1990, as it has been considered as a powerful driving force to improve the effectiveness and standard of national health systems and to promote empowerment and equity by reducing the unmet demands of the community (Collins et al. 2003a, b; WHO 2008a; Costa-Font 2012). The World Bank (2004) highlights tripartite dynamics of decentralization between service users (clients), citizens (people) and institutional systems to be able to make services responsive to the needs of people by making government closer to citizens and closer to services.

Decentralization is in fact a catch-all description rather than a definitive reform mechanism in health, as it is not one concept in itself but is highly contested. It is therefore important to focus on what type of decentralization is being addressed and how it affects health system design and functioning. It is, however, interesting to point out that the most appropriate level of decentralization in the health system is an important unresolved policy debate (Robalino et al. 2001; Peckham et al. 2005; Kurk and Freeman 2008; Siddiqi et al. 2009). In addition, several authors have also noted that very 'little attention has been paid to the measurement of decentralization in health services, as opposed to the relatively greater amount of literature available about the effects of decentralization on government size, economic growth', equity and performance (Smith 1997; Jimenez and Smith 2005, p. 3; Peckham et al. 2005).

The notion of the decentralization policies is, however, to develop a new type of health-care organisation that would allocate some degree of 'spaces' to local authorities or local governments to assess, analyse and then plan and deliver (action) appropriate health-care services, keeping people at the centre of their policies (Bossert 1996; Peckham et al. 2005), i.e. nothing about us without us (Werner 1998). The World Bank (n.d., p.x.) states that for two important reasons we failed to measure the effects of decentralization on health sector outcomes: first, 'how these benefits can be realised', if any, and in what context and, second, 'specific impact of different health system reforms are not well understood'. Similarly, Wollmann (2008) also argues two important 'deficits' to make the decentralization reform inevitable: (a) democratic deficit (poor accountability and transparency prevails in decision-making at the local levels) and (b) performance deficit (local authorities have consistently failed to address wider determinants (socio-economic, political and environmental)).

Analysis of decentralization policies in many developing parts of the world may draw on similar principles and theoretical frameworks as decentralization in the UK or USA, but they are different due to their different socio-economic and political landscapes. In the USA, for example, Medicaid (health insurance) is one of the programmes for which important elements of federal authority have been devolved to the states; in the UK, the English National Health Service (NHS) is one of the basic responsibilities of the new Scottish and Welsh parliaments; and in Spain and Italy, legislative powers have been combined with an augmented fiscal autonomy in health care (Jiménez and Smith 2004, p. 2). In many parts of the world, the motives of decentralization of health services by different funding agencies, such as the World Bank and UNDP, vary, and they influence recipient's spending patterns and budgetary process (Atkinson et al. 2000; Rubio and Smith 2004; WHO 2008b). The World Bank (2004), for example, noted some donors interfere directly with the design and deliver of public services:

> 'First, donors may support only capital spending (construction) and expect the government to supply complementary inputs (staff, maintenance). Governments often fail to finance the complementary inputs. Second, donors may fund projects that governments are not interested in. This contradicts ownership. Third, donors may set targets for the share of spending in particular sectors as conditions for flow. Fourth, donors may give aid to a priority sector and assume that government spending from its own resources remain unchanged' (p. 204).

Decentralization is fundamentally 'politically motivated, and consequently much of the literature has stressed the advantages—service access and responsiveness and limitations of the sub-national (district/sub-district) provision of health services' (Jimenez and Smith 2005, p.3; Rubio 2006). There is not much strong evidence prevailing, for example, 'countries with a more decentralised health system experience better health outcomes' (Conyers 1986; Manor 1997a, b; Shah et al. 2004; Jimenez and Smith 2005, p.13; Prieto and Saez 2006; Rubio 2006; Kurk and Freedman 2008). Therefore the 'means and ends' of decentralization are different both rhetorically and in practice. In the case of health care, it is often pursued with the motive of political, technical and financial purposes—sometimes technical means of improving the effectiveness of management and service delivery (WHO 2008a); politically, seeking community participation, power and autonomy (WHO 2008a, p.1; WHO 2008b); and fiscally as a means of cost-effectiveness and cost-efficiency (Saltman et al. 1997, 2003; Agrawal et al. 1999; WHO 2004, 2007; World Bank 2004a, b). It is, therefore, important to set out the nature of decentralization—focusing more on the elements of what is often parcelled up as decentralization. This includes institutional reform, political change, autonomy and accountability.

Activity 1

What are the organisational polices and professional opportunities and barriers to implementing decentralization in health services?

Typology of Decentralization

Decentralization is a complex term to define as it not only brings different paradigms and perspectives into place but also takes many forms and dimensions including labelling and labels (Fig. 1.1). This is complex in nature—as Omar (2002, pp. 25–26) argues 'no country conforms to any single category of decentralization, but manifests multiple elements of the different forms of decentralization at the same time'—within countries and even within sectors; second, there is clearly some overlap between/among their concepts and interpretations.

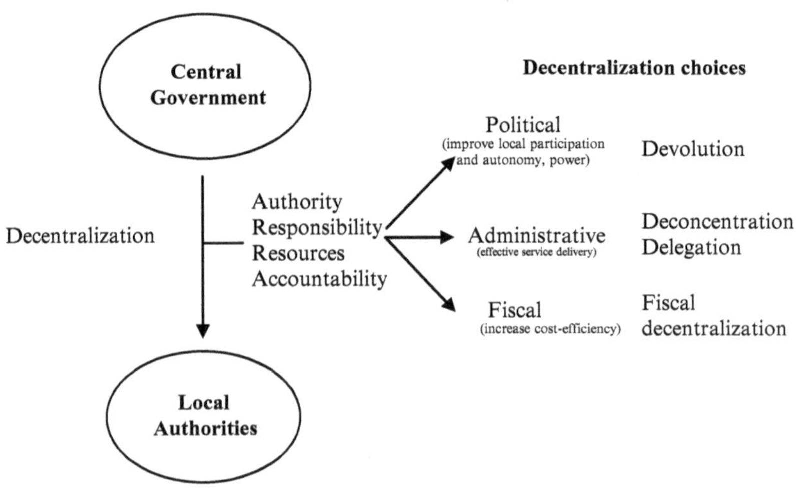

Fig. 1.1 Typology of decentralization [Source: Saltman et al. (2007), Cohen and Peterson (1999)]

Different authors review decentralization in different forms and levels. Treisman (2002, p.14), for example, views decentralization in six dimensions: vertical decentralization (based on the number of tiers), decision-making decentralization (space provided to make political decisions at the local level), appointment decentralization (whether local authorities have the right to make any executive appointments), electoral decentralization (nature of local authorities/officials are elected), fiscal decentralization (sharing/generating revenues and taxes) and personal decentralization (roles of local employees in total government). Meanwhile Rondinelli (1981, 1989), a renowned author and internationally established subject expert, offers three types of decentralization, i.e. political decentralization (devolution), administrative decentralization (deconcentration and delegation) and fiscal decentralization.

1. Political Form of Decentralization (Devolution)
   Decentralised systems bring more accessibility to political movements and minority groups in their attempts to influence politics—this is particularly important to the national and international contexts where there are ethnically divided societies, and political exclusion can have serious polarising effects (Hadenius 2003, p.1; also see World Bank 1997; Grindle 2000). Inman and Rubinfeld (1997) argue that political decentralization would help to map local people's needs and interests while making decisions at policy levels.

   Political decentralization is often called devolution, where central government transfers authority and responsibility to local authorities (quasi-autonomous units of local government) for decision-making, finance and management. This approach is also called an extensive form of decentralization, as this often transfers responsibilities to that unit (municipalities or districts, provinces or villages) who are elected from their community, can raise their own revenues and have a great amount of decision space at the local discretion. In Rondinelli's (1989) view, local government will have established legal boundaries to exercise their power and authority to deliver public services. The aim of political decentralization is to promote people's participation in local planning and decision-making. This approach is often called an institutionalised form of strengthening democratic decentralization (see Ribot 2002; Kassibo 2002; Cohen and Peterson 1999).

   Characteristics

- Radical form of restructuring/reforming health services.
- There is little or no direct control by the central government—local government or local authorities are autonomous and independent.
- Normally there are clear legal and geographical boundaries of local bodies (LBs), within which they perform their functions and exercise devolved authority.
- The local governments to which the power and responsibilities have been devolved are perceived as government units.
- Granted few revenue-raising powers.
- On the basis of the concept of reciprocity, a coordinated relationship between the central and local government takes place for their mutual benefit.
- Decision-makers are elected representatives accountable to voters who participate in other ways in the political life of local communities or regions.

- Effectiveness will often be determined by four sets of supportive conditions: political and administrative, organisational and institutional, behavioural and psychological and the availability of resources.
  Source: Cheema and Rondinelli 1983; Smith 1985, p.11; Mills et al. 1990.

  It is, therefore, important to acknowledge that to make a successful 'transition' of transferring authority and responsibility between the different levels/tiers of government, three important components should interplay—political, fiscal and economic aspects.

2. Administrative Form of Decentralization (Deconcentration and Delegation)
   Administrative decentralization relates to the process of how defined political institutions would make collective decisions to bring distributive outcomes utilising both fiscal and regulatory mechanisms. As Litvack et al. (1998) argue, political decisions aim 'to devolve powers from central government, for example, can only get translated into actual powers being shifted if supranational governments have the fiscal, political, and administrative capacity to manage this responsibility' (p.6).

   Deconcentration—a form of administrative decentralization where central government disperse responsibilities of certain services to their own regional/local branches. This however does not involve transfer of authority and responsibility to the local government and is unlikely to lead to the potential benefits or pitfalls (Regmi et al. 2009). Though there may be some 'downward' accountability (to service users, etc.) built into their functions, their primary responsibilities are to represent the central government and to deliver public services on its behalf (World Bank & United Cites and Local Governments, 2008, p.306). Indeed, much of the developing world—East Asia and Eastern Europe—adopt this approach as a form of decentralization, as in many government systems there is no legally separate identity of local independent government and regional/local branches which are used to make services effective and efficient. Litvack et al. (1998) suggest deconcentration is sometimes used to deliver certain functions in federal countries when there are certain strong government systems.

   Delegation—the extent to which central government transfers authority and responsibility to local governments or semi-autonomous institutions, often called 'parastatal organisations', for making public services more effective. One argument is that this form of decentralization applies when local governments or semi-autonomous institutions are not solely dependent on the control or command of central government—that means local governments have some degree of space to make decisions independently. As Bossert (1998) suggests, such a form of decentralization could also be viewed as a 'principal (central government)—agent (local governments/semi-auto institutions)' approach.

   Characteristics

- Deconcentration entails the redistribution or 'handing over' of some administrative responsibilities to lower units of central government without transferring any authority to make independent decisions (Kassibo, 2002).

- Involves the transfer of administrative rather than political responsibility, and it has been the form of decentralization most frequently used in developing nations (Mills et al. 1990).
- It is usually regarded as a weaker form of decentralization because downward accountability is not well established, unlike in the democratic or political forms. In certain cases of delegation, certain responsibilities are transferred to organisations which are outside the bureaucratic structure and are indirectly controlled by the central government (Cohen and Peterson 1999).

3. Fiscal Form of Decentralization

   The process of making appropriate decisions through the defined nature and form of taxes and approaches. Several studies have noted that decentralization with local and central regions able to decide about financial matters as per the nation's own requirements brings about better health outcomes (Litvack et al. 1998). In addition, it is important to note that there should be a strong local network of professionals who offer support with their skills and capacities to assess, identify and analyse appropriate problems and concerns (Kocia 2008).

   Characteristics

- Fiscal decentralization aims to bring about the 'transfer of the resources necessary for the exercise of the transferred powers and responsibilities' (World Bank & United Cites and Local Governments 2008, p. 306).

In some literatures, privatisation, deregulation and divestment are presented as forms of market decentralization. Privatisation entails the 'transfers of functions to the private sectors including planning and administration, previously held by public institutions' (World Bank & United Cites and Local Governments 2008, p.306), but usually they are excluded from decentralization typologies, as Ribot (2002) notes that privatised markets mostly operate for profit motives rather than public accountability, and most importantly, a greater amount of authority and responsibility would remain in the centre (also see Bossert 1996; Green and Matthias 1997). However, several authors (Litvac et al. 1998; Litvac and Jessica 2005; Mills et al. 1990) equally argue that decentralization is not necessarily confined only to the public sector—it may happen with the voluntary sectors whose motive may not be profit-seeking, for example, non-governmental organisations, trade unions and professional bodies. Green and Matthias (1997) view this group as defined as 'formal organisations, which have corporate objectives concerned with humanitarian aims concerning groups outside the direct control of government' (p. 7). Nevertheless, both devolution and deconcentration are taken as means of pushing forward the angel of privatisation (Slater 1989).

Activity 2

Can you identify any factors which help or hinder the translation of decentralization of health sector policy into practice?

Opportunities and Challenges of Decentralization

As the nature of decentralization is complex, thereby its opportunities and significance to practice are complex too. Litvack et al. (1998) discuss three important implications: First, decentralization is a process of negotiation between central and local tiers of governments through mobilisation and allocation of resources, which as a result might have positive effects from service delivery to poverty reduction. Second, understanding of institutional content (knowledge), context and process of decentralization is paramount. There is a need to understand the driving forces and the stakeholders involved. Third, there is still limited information—either non-existent or conflicting—on how and in what context, if any, decentralization does or does not work. Similarly, Crook and Manor (1998) also note that the 'outcomes of a decentralization policy will depend not just on the relative weights of devolution and deconcentration in the institutional and fiscal structures, but also on their combination with two other important elements: the kind of legitimation and accountability adopted (e.g. participatory, electoral) and the principles according to which the areas (and hence size and character) of a decentralised authority are determined' (p. 2).

Health sector decentralization advocates point out its various perceived benefits (Mills et al. 1990; Conn et al. 1996). Since the 1990s, management of health services has shifted from the costly curative model, to become more promotive and preventive, where community or service users are actively involved in planning and management, including sharing benefits through restructuring of power between the central and local authorities (Mills et al. 1990; Mills 1994; Chambers 1983, 1995, 1997; WHO 2008b).

Mills et al. (1990, p.142), however, highlight key promises of decentralization in health care:

- Organise a more rational and unified health service on the basis of geographical and administrative areas that will be able to address local people's health-care preferences.
- Involve local communities in the management of their own health.
- Reduce duplication of services, particularly at the secondary and tertiary levels of health care, by relating responsibilities to defined catchment populations.
- Reduce inequalities between regions and between rural and urban areas.
- Integrate service activities of government and non-governmental and private health organisations.
- Reduce centralised control over local administrative matters.
- Encourage greater community financing and control over primary health-care facilities and staff.
- Inter-sectoral coordination between the health sector and other sectors, particularly at the local levels.

Success Factors of Decentralization

Decentralization is a complex phenomenon, and it does embed with different socio-economic, political and institutional factors as well as countries' own health systems and infrastructure. Therefore there is more than one factor to determine the success of any decentralization reform. Some of the important points as enablers or drivers to make decentralization in health services successful are:

- A strong and sustained political will and commitment to delegate authority and stop encroaching on authority already delegated.
- Improved capacity of local authorities needs to be appraised and necessary training and support provided so that all their executions are based on informed decisions.
- Redefine the new and strategic role of various levels of central authorities, and restructure them accordingly so as to avoid ambiguities in discharging functions.
- Strengthen the process development—development of strategies, standards, norms and performance indicators.
- Strengthen local—district—or provisional health systems management.
- Develop appropriate analytical frameworks to study the achievements attained through the assessment of the performance-based health outcomes.
- Systems of accountability to be able to measure the effectiveness of local government functions on people using an appropriate and responsive legal and institutional framework.
- Establish a high-level task force involving all stakeholders engaging in the process of monitoring utility-based research on local health systems, introducing new innovative choices for better health performance in local authorities.
- Widen the decision space for the local bodies not only to exercise power and authority but also to execute functions tailored to local needs and demands. Source: WHO (2007, p.2)

Challenges

Though there are some promising outcomes of the effect of decentralization in health services, (re)distribution of authorities, responsibilities and resources are never exempt from controversy (Costa-Font 2012, p.252). Several studies warn that decentralization may result in the inequitable distribution of resources or bring challenges related to insufficient human resource capacity (Kolehmainen-Aitken 1999;

Lubben et al. 2002). Several authors (Standing 1997; Kaufman and Jing 2002) rather reveal negative outcomes between the association of health sector reforms, privatisation and health outcomes. Similarly, a review of the literature on decentralization in Asia noted that decentralization of health systems had a negative impact on health, though the existing evidences are insufficient to support this assertion (Collins et al. 2003a, b) and a number of challenges have been noted—limited authority and autonomy, poor institutional mechanisms and a weak level of trust among actors. It is clear from a review of pertinent literatures on the impact of decentralization that a number of tensions still exist among researchers. Some assume that decentralization is 'good in itself' without explaining why it is desirable (Bossert and Beauvais 2002; Collins et al. 2003a, b). Others see 'decentralization as a means (or process) of achieving specific objectives rather than an end (or outcome)' in itself (Peckham et al. 2005, p.38).

Therefore, it can be argued that decentralization is one of the most widely debated topics among politicians, bureaucrats and donor communities (Saltman et al. 2007). WHO (2007) adds that though decentralization may create more power and space for the local authorities, arguably this process might equally create some monopolisation of power by certain elites—often the consequences of centralised political and administrative structures (Hadenius 2003). Costa-Font (2012) discussed several myths about the effects of decentralization on health services, i.e. regional inequalities, privatisation, inefficacity and lower productivity which might be emerged from the assumptions and speculations rather than the empirical evidences. It is therefore important to acknowledge two important facts: first, it has been consistently noted that inappropriate design of decentralization would have negative impacts on health service delivery (Gilson et al. 1994; Kolehmainen-Aitken and Newbrander 1997); second, a lack of reliable analytical frameworks brings some challenges to effectively measuring the effects of decentralization in health at appropriate levels (Bossert 1997).

Activity 3

To what extent has decentralization contributed to making health services effective, efficient, equal and accessible? What other factors were involved?'

Conclusion

This chapter discussed the concept of decentralization as a process within policy and political options rather than a truly 'dependent or independent' variable or product (Bossert 1998; Peckham et al. 2005). Though decentralization offers inspiring vision, it is often challenging to translate its forms and mechanisms into practice as it embeds a number of assumptions, speculations, contradictions, tensions and challenges. This also highlights that success of decentralization in public services—health determines not only the degree and the extent of fiscal, political and administrative choices and how best they interplay but also institutional development, better information systems and strengthening better capacities and capabilities of both central and local peoples including civil societies to bring sectoral performance and a wide range of outcomes. In addition, health reforms should link to better planning of human resource and stewardship by governments and should provide technical capacity and appropriate information systems. Though the participation of the private sector in health has not been a well-researched theme, it is equally important to investigate its wider role to increase the efficiency, quality and effectiveness of the health sector. Most importantly, government should have a strong political will to reform the health sector, as many nations across the world would have still frequent changes of government; political instability and poor citizen empowerment are the major pitfalls of a successful decentralization.

Activity 4

In what ways can decentralization be described as 'means'? In what ways can it be described as 'ends'?

Further Discussion

- Which form(s) or type(s) of decentralization would you favour in your specialised field and why?
- To what extent do you agree with this statement? 'All services do not need to be decentralised in the same way or to the same degree.' Discuss.
- Whether decentralised systems devolution would be the best option to bring services closer to the public while making services effective and efficient or whether centralised government would still equally impact positively if resources and capacity at the local level were raised and improved. Discuss.

Recommended Reading

Burns, D., Hambleton, R., & Hoggett, P. (1994). *The politics of decentralization: Revitalising local democracy*. Basingstoke: McMillan.

Useful textbook, which focuses mostly on market and competition into public services from the neighbourhood perspective.

Cohen, J. M., & Peterson, S. B. (1999). *Administrative decentralization: Strategies for developing countries*. Oakwood: Kumari Press.

Readable textbook, which has been recommended for some PG management courses in some universities, both in developed and developing countries. This book highlights the 'administrative' aspect of decentralization, and draws experiences mostly from developing countries.

Saltman, R. B., Bankauskaite, V., & Vrangbaek, K. (2007). *Decentralization in health care*. London: OUP.

Popular reading resource on 'decentralization and healthcare' from the experience of EU contexts.

Bardhan, P., & Mookherjee, D. (2006). *Decentralization and local governance in developing countries: A comparative perspective*. London: MIT Press.

Useful textbook, which mostly draws on experience from the economic viewpoint of decentralization. This book may be beneficial at strengthening the capacity, through education and training, and capability of the workforce to contribute to public services reform and development.

References

Atkinson, S., Medeiros, R. L., Oliveira, P. H., & de Almeida, R. D. (2000). Going down to the local: Incorporating social organisation and political culture into assessments of decentralised health care. *Social Science and Medicine, 4*, 619–636.

Bienen, H., Kapur, D., & Parks, J. (1990). Decentralization in Nepal. *World Development, 18*(1), 61–75.

Bossert, T. (1996). Decentralization. In K. Jonovsky (Ed.), *Decentralization in health policy and system development: An agenda for research* (pp. 147–159). Geneva: WHO.

Bossert, T. (1997). *Decentralization of health systems: Decision space, innovation and performance*. Boston, MA: Harvard School of Public Health. Accessed August 15, 2013, from http://www.hsph.harvard.edu/ihsg/publications/pdf/No-54.PDF.

Bossert, T. (1998). Analyzing the decentralization of health systems in developing countries: Decision space, innovation and performance. *Social Science and Medicine, 47*, 1513–1527.

Chambers, R. (1983). *Rural development: Putting the last first*. Essex, UK: Longman.

Chambers, R. (1995). Paradigm shifts and practice of participatory research and development. In N. Nelson & S. Wright (Eds.), *Power and participatory development: Theory and practice*. London: Intermediate Technology Publications.

Chambers, R. (1997). *Whose reality counts?* London: Intermediate Technology Publications.

Cheema, G., & Rondinelli, D. (1983). *Decentralization and development: Policy implementation in developing countries*. London: Sage Publications.

Cohen, J., & Peterson, S. (1999). *Administrative decentralization: Strategies for developing countries*. USA: Kumarian Press.

Collins, C., Omar, M., Adhikari, D., Emmel, N., Dhakal, M. R., & Thapa, D. (2003a). *Developing health sector decentralization in Nepal: Collaborative policy development*. Leeds, UK: GON-DFID, DSHP.

Collins, C., Omar, M., Adhikari, D., Emmel, N., Dhakal, M. R., & Thapa, D. (2003b). *Developing a project for effective health sector decentralization in Nepal*. Nepal: British Council-DIFD, DHSP.

Conyers, D. (1986). Decentralization and development: A framework for analysis. *Community Development Journal, 21*(2), 88–100.

Gilson, L., Kilima, P., & Tanner, M. (1994). Local government decentralization and the health sector in Tanzania. *Public Administration and Development, 14*, 451–477.

Jimenez, D., & Smith, P. C. (2005). *Decentralization of health care and its impact on health outcomes. No. 2005/10*. York, UK: Department of Economics and Related Studies, University of York.

Kassibo, B. (2002). *Participatory management and democratic decentralization management of the Samori forest in Babye commune, Mopti region, Mali*. Accessed October 15, 2013, from http://dlc.dlib.indiana.edu/dlc/bitstream/handle/10535/1375/kassibob210502.pdf

Kaufman, J., & Jing, F. (2002). Privatisation of health services and the reproductive health of rural Chinese women. *Reproductive Health Matters, 10*(20), 108–116.

Kocia, A. (2008). Fiscal systems competition. *Argumenta Oeconomica, 1*(20), 31–44.

Kolehmainen-Aitken, R. (1999). *Implementation and integration of reproductive health services in a decentralized system: Myths and realities about the decentralization of health systems*. Newton, MA: Management Sciences for Health.

Kolehmainen-Aitken, R., & Newbrander, W. (1997). *Decentralizing the management of Health and Family Planning Programs*. Newton, MA: Management Sciences for Health.

Kurk, M. E., & Freedman, L. P. (2008). Assessing health system performance in developing countries: A review of literature. *Health Policy, 85*, 263–276.

Manor, J. (1997a). *Explaining the popularity of decentralization*. Washington, DC: World Bank.
Manor, J. (1997b). *The promise and limitations of decentralization*. Washington, DC: World Bank.
Mills, A. (1994). Decentralization and accountability in the health sector from an international perspective: What are the choices? *Public Administration and Development, 14*, 281–292.
Mills, A., Vaughan, J., Smith, D., & Tabibzadeh, I. (1990). *Health system decentralization: Concepts, issues and country experience*. Geneva: WHO.
Prieto, D. C., & Saez, M. P. (2006). *Decentralization and health care outcomes: An empirical analysis within the European Union*. Accessed August 22, 2013, from http://www.fedea.es/pub/eee/eee220.pdf
Regmi, K., Naidoo, J., Pilkington, P., & Greer, A. (2009). Decentralization and district health services in Nepal: Understanding the views of service users and service providers. *Journal of Public Health, 32*(3), 406–417.
Robalino, D. A., Picazo, O., & Voetberg, A. (2001). *Does fiscal decentralization improve health outcomes? Evidence from a cross-country analysis* (World Bank Policy Research Working Paper). Washington, DC: World Bank, Kenya Country Team.
Rondinelli, D. A., (1981). Government decentralization in comparative perspective: The theory and practice in developing countries. *Public Administration, XIVII*, 133–145.
Rondinelli, A. (1989). Decentralising public services in developing countries: Issues and opportunities. *Journal of Social, Political and Economic Status, 14*, 77–97.
Rubio, D. J. (2006). *Decentralization and its impact on health and inequity in health: Some theoretical considerations and implications to Canada*. York, UK: University of York.
Rubio, D. J., & Smith, P. C. (2004, May). *Decentralization of health care and its impact on health outcomes*. Paper presented to conference XXIV Jornadas de Economia de la Salud, El Escorial.
Saltman, R. B., Bankauskaite, V., & Vrangbaek, K. (2007). *Decentralization in health care*. London: OUP.
Saltman, R. B., & Figureras, J. (1997). *European health care reform: Analysis of current strategies* (WHO Regional Publication, European Series No. 72). Copenhagen: WHO.
School of Oriental and African Studies. (SOAS). (2009). *Decentralization and local governance: Course introduction and overview*. London: University of London.
Shah, A., Thomson, T., & Zou, H. (2004). *The impact of decentralization on service delivery, corruption, fiscal management and growth in developing market economies: A synthesis of empirical evidence*. Accessed August 18, 2013, from http://www.ifo.de/pls/guestci/download/CESifo%20DICE%20Report%202004/CESifo%20DICE%20Report%201/2004/dicereport104-forum2.pdf
Siddiqi, S., Masud, T. I., Nishtar, S., Peters, D. H., Sabri, B., Bile, K. M., et al. (2009). Framework for assessing governance of the health systems in developing countries: Gateway to good governance. *Health Policy, 90*, 13–25.
Smith, B. C. (1985). *Decentralization: The territorial dimension of the state*. London: George Allen and Unwin Publications.
Smith, B. C. (1997). The decentralization of health care in developing countries: Organizational options. *Public Administration and Development, 17*, 399–412.
United Nations Development Programme. (1999). *Report on global workshop on UNDP/MIT decentralised governance research project*. Amman, Jordon: Author.
Work, R. (2002, July). '*Overview of decentralization worldwide: A stepping stone to improved governance and human development*'. *Federalism: the future of decentralising states?* 2nd International Conference on Decentralization, Manila, Philippines.
World Bank & United Cities and Local Governments. (2008). *Decentralization and local democracy in the world: First global report*. Barcelona: United Cites and Local Governments.
World Health Organization. (2008a). *Decentralization and health system and its management*. Accessed July 27, 2013, from http://www.nep.searo.who.int/LinkFiles/Home_Dececentralization_of_Health_System.pdf
World Health Organization. (2008b). *The world health report 2008: Primary health care now more than ever*. Geneva: WHO.

Chapter 2
Health Systems and Decentralization

Patrick Tobi and Krishna Regmi

Abstract Health systems are comprised of many programmes, functions and interventions tailored to improve people's health. All health systems share certain common features, such as the ways they are organised and financed and deliver services. Providing better health systems means maintaining people's good health, fairness of financial contribution and delivering responsive health-care services to those who need them. This chapter provides a global overview of health systems with an emphasis on decentralised systems in low- and middle-income countries. Examples from different country systems and circumstances are discussed to provide a real context and draw attention to variations in system configuration.

By the End of the Chapter, You Will Be Able to

- *Understand the importance of health systems.*
- *Identify the broad features that characterise health systems.*
- *Describe the functions and goals of health systems.*
- *Understand the rationale and challenges of health systems reform and decentralization.*

P. Tobi
Institute for Health and Human Development, University of East London,
Water Lane, London, UK
e-mail: p.tobi@uel.ac.uk

K. Regmi (✉)
Department of Clinical Education and Leadership, Faculty of Health & Social Sciences - Institute for Health Research, University of Bedfordshire, Putteridge Bury Campus,
Room 32, Luton LU2 8LE, UK
e-mail: krishna.regmi@beds.ac.uk

K. Regmi (ed.), *Decentralizing Health Services: A Global Perspective*,
DOI 10.1007/978-1-4614-9071-5_2, © Springer Science+Business Media New York 2014

Introduction

After many decades of approaching health from a disease-specific focus, the attention of many organisations involved in global health shifted to a more systemic perspective (Hafner and Shiffman 2013). The 2000 World Health Report was dedicated to the topic of health systems (WHO 2000). It examined characteristics of health systems around the world and provided conceptual insights into the multifaceted factors that explain how health systems perform and how the performance can be measured. Since the release of the report, there has been sustained interest in understanding how health systems contribute to the health of the populations they serve. Again in 2010, the focus of the World Health Report was on health financing, a major component of the health system (WHO 2010a).

Yet, even though there is universal acknowledgement of their role in health, there is still some uncertainty, even amongst health professionals, about what exactly health systems are and what they do. Opinions appear to be influenced by people's understanding of health and health care itself. These viewpoints have been to a large extent influenced by a medical perspective in which health is seen as the absence of illness and health care as the provision of services to treat illness and maintain health.

Another influence on our understanding stems from the fact that health systems are by nature complex, but attempts to explain them often end up reducing their complexity to more elemental processes. According to Simon (1982), this reductionist and linear approach creates 'bounded rationality', whereby we construct a representation of the health system that is bounded or limited by our inability to comprehend and analyse all its component parts and interrelationships. In essence, we simplify the system to the sum of its individual parts. Atun (2012) draws attention to this complexity, highlighting that many well-intentioned policies and managerial decisions aimed at improving health systems fail because 'too often the tools used for analysing health systems and the heuristics used to generate managerial decisions are too simplistic for health systems that are complex'.

This chapter aims to provide a global overview of health systems. It describes their characteristics, configuration and boundaries and highlights the different ways well-functioning health systems contribute to improving health. It further examines decentralization in the context of health system reform.

What Is a Health System?

It has long been a common misconception to think of the public sector service delivery system as the health system. It is not surprising therefore that the terms 'health system' and 'health sector' have often been used interchangeably and interpreted to mean the actions of the government or State. Such a view excludes the services provided by the non-State sector, i.e. the health professionals and facilities in the private and voluntary sectors. Again, when people talk of the health system, they often describe it in terms of health-care delivery. The two are not the same; the latter is part of the wider health system and refers to the provision or delivery of health services. Contemporary understanding of the health system is more encompassing and sees it in terms of linked networks of actors and actions. This understanding adopts a broader perspective that incorporates all sectors—public, private and voluntary. The central message is that an acknowledgement of these broader influences, together with the complex interactions and linkages amongst them, is critical for understanding the health system.

Perhaps the most widely recognised characterisation of health systems comes from the World Health Organization. It defined the health system to include all the activities whose primary purpose is to promote, restore or maintain health (WHO 2000; p. 5). The health system can also be described as consisting of all the organisations, institutions and resources that are devoted to producing health actions. What is included within these boundaries? It embraces formal health services as well as community care, home care, self care and traditional health services. It includes the full range of players engaged in the provision and financing of health services such as the public, non-profit and for-profit private sectors, as well as international and bilateral donors, foundations and voluntary organisations involved in funding or implementing health activities. It also includes efforts to influence the determinants of health as well as more direct health improvement and promotion activities (WHO 2010b, p. vi).

The key factor in deciding whether a resource is part of the health system or not depends on whether the *primary* purpose of the resource is concerned with promoting, restoring or maintaining health. The primary purpose distinguishes activities within the boundaries of the system from those whose principal purpose is something other than health but may have a secondary health benefit. There are many ways to promote and sustain health that lie outside the confines of the health system, for instance, activities within the social care and general education sectors. These can have benefits for health but are not considered part of the health system.

Within our understanding of the goal of the health system as being to maintain and improve health, we can think of it as comprising three main parts (Zakus and Bhattacharyya 2007, p. 278):

- The totality of the required resources, including human, mechanical, material and financial
- The formal and informal organisation interactions or conversions of these resources in the provision of direct services to individuals and populations to help them maintain good health status or improve their health status when it is perceived in need, from either disease, physical disability or trauma
- The final product of health, which can vary in definition but is commonly understood as the state of complete physical, mental and social (including spiritual) well-being or the ability to live one's life in a manner that is compatible with achieving one's social and individual goals

Why Do Health Systems Matter?

We mentioned in the introduction to the chapter that attention had shifted from disease-specific initiatives to health system approaches to health improvement. Piette et al. (2012) argue that one reason this shift has occurred is because difficulties in achieving health targets, such as the Millennium Development Goals, and growing consumer demand for care have forced health policymakers to look for innovative ways to deliver better health outcomes whilst controlling service costs. Part of that innovation has been demonstrated in the development of holistic ways of thinking that are required when working from a health systems perspective (Atun 2012).

Another motivation is that the current environment is one in which international and sectoral boundaries have become progressively more permeable (Smith and Hanson 2011). The result of this is that partnership working has increased as different services, organisations, sectors and even countries acknowledge that the scale of the challenges they face is beyond the capacity of any one health provider. They recognise that improving population health requires joined up effort and can only be effectively tackled by the different parts of the health system working together.

Health systems must do many things at the same time—for instance, address diverse population needs, provide high-quality services and improve training and support for health-care workers. It is therefore important that the system functions properly. Disrupted or fractured health systems have become a common feature of the global political landscape owing to social and political instability in many regions of the world. Initially such instability was observed largely in countries that had experienced protracted military conflict or large scale disasters such as Afghanistan, Mozambique, Rwanda, Sudan, Angola, the Democratic Republic of the Congo and Somalia.

However, the current global economic meltdown has produced a different driver for disruption in countries such as Greece, Ireland Estonia, the Czech Republic and Spain (Thomas et al. 2012). Concerns about the potential impact of the financial crisis on the ability of countries to achieve health system goals led the World Health Organization's Regional Committee to adopt the 2009 resolution *Health in times of global economic crisis*: *implications for the WHO European Region* (EUR/RC59/R3a) (Mladovsky et al. 2012).

A well-functioning health system achieves good health, organises and uses resources efficiently, is responsive to the expectations of users and protects them from unfair financial expenditure (Box 2.1). For this reason, many global health initiatives now routinely incorporate attention to health systems strengthening within their portfolio of support.

Box 2.1 Importance of Health Systems

A well-functioning health system responds in a balanced way to a population's needs and expectations by:

- Improving the health status of individuals, families and communities
- Defending the population against what threatens its health
- Protecting people against the financial consequences of ill health
- Providing equitable access to people-centred care
- Making it possible for people to participate in decisions affecting their health and the health system

Source: WHO 2010b, p1

Functions and Goals of the Health System

A general way to describe any system is by looking at what goes into it (inputs), what makes up it's parts (structure), what happens within it (processes) and what effects it produces (outputs). Applying this framework to the health system, inputs will include such things as human resources, technology, financing and equipment, while structure is represented by the organisation of public health infrastructure, hospitals, clinics and extended care facilities. Health system processes are the operations of different departments and bodies and the provision of services. Outputs consist of outcomes, quality, access and costs (Busse and Wismar 2002).

However, health system experts are not just interested in descriptive models of the health system. Rather, they want to characterise the system in more analytical ways that aid understanding of how component parts of the system can be manipulated to ensure that it is functioning well and has the capacity to achieve its goals. Therefore, any effort to deconstruct the health system is intended not merely to identify its component parts but to define them from the viewpoint of their functionality, i.e. contribution to achieving the goals of the system.

There are various elements of health systems utilised across the world. Roemer (1991), for example, has highlighted five common categories appropriate to many countries' health systems: (a) production of resources (staff, commodities, facilities), (b) planning and organisation of health programmes (inter- and intra-organisational collaborations), (c) economic support mechanism (sources of funds, tax, user fees), (d) management styles (planning, monitoring and regulation) and (e) nature of delivery of health services (primary, secondary and tertiary services; target populations; etc.). Recently, the World Health Organization (2006, 2007) identified six critical health system components that need to be in good working order to render equitable and sustained improved services. These are leadership and governance/stewardship (originally called policy), financing, human resources, supply systems, service management and information and monitoring systems. They are described in greater detail in the box below.

Box 2.2 Health System Functions

1. **Leadership and Governance/Stewardship**. Originally termed policy by the WHO (2006), this function refers to the strategic direction set by senior policymakers to protect public health and safety, control corruption and contribute to effective leadership of the country's health sector. It includes the legislative, regulatory and policymaking processes, incentives and sanction mechanisms, adjudication systems and coordination/harmonisation with other donors or public sector actors to ensure equitable and sustained health services.

(continued)

Box 2.2 (continued)

2. **Health financing** refers to the mobilisation, collection, pooling and distribution of health resources to improve their allocation and utilisation; maximise outcomes, equity and health status; and protect citizens from catastrophic health expenditures.
3. **Human resources for health** (**HRH**) refers to the health workforce and includes all the different cadre of health workers such as nurses, doctors, medical clerks, ward attendants and community outreach workers. HRH takes up the major part of the health system's budget, accounting for about 70 % of health-care costs in most countries. It not only is the most expensive component of the health system but has been identified as the single most important ingredient in the amount and quality of health-care provision.
4. **Supply systems** refers to the national system to provide drugs, medical products, vaccines, commodities and technologies. It includes drug policy development, registration and regulation, quality assurance/control mechanisms as well as drug and commodity selection, quantification, procurement, warehousing and distribution.
5. **Service management** refers to improving the organisation, management and quality of services. The organisation of services is concerned with the development and implementation of models of care that promote effective delivery of high-quality services at the appropriate level (community, primary, secondary, tertiary) and reduce segmentation of care. Activities may also focus on referral networks or systems between service levels and mechanisms for quality improvement. Management takes place at many different levels in the health system, and weaknesses in management can make services less effective and waste resources.
6. **Information and monitoring systems** refers to the collection and analysis of accurate routine health information for management decision-making. This includes development of national surveillance systems and surveys, and the design of programme reporting forms and standard medical record forms for accurate reporting of health services statistics.

Source: WHO 2007, p3; WHO 2006, p4

The relationship between the system functions and goals is illustrated in Fig. 2.1.

Health System Reform

Health reforms are the processes or means of organisational and financial changes based on social and political values (Gilson, 1997). There are different approaches to reforming health systems across the world: top-down, bottom-up, vertical,

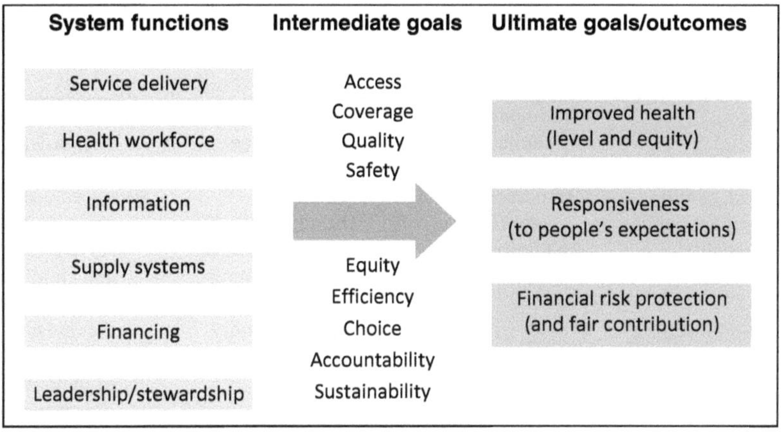

Fig. 2.1 Adapted from WHO (2007), p.3

horizontal and so on. The most common approach advocated by World Health Organization (2005) in many developing nations is the primary health-care approach. Dekker (1994) notes there are two main approaches to reform of health services, particularly from the perspective of a European context: first, a bit of public health with the approach of health for all and, second, more of a health service-focused approach. The first approach relates to the improvement of efficiency of health services through changing institutional administration, financial and organisational aspects, which appears a more holistic system approach.

Several authors (Saltman 1994; Leighton 1996) viewed health system reform in terms of three aspects: finance (Europe—more competition amongst private firms versus revenue raising in Africa), production (Europe, regulation; Africa, alternative modes of health-care delivery) and allocation (through contracts in Europe and reallocation in Africa). Health systems relate to all aspects of organisations, institutions and resources that are required to ensure that appropriate services are offered and rendered accessible to the target people in the form of system: (a) inputs, resources (human capital, infrastructure, equipment, medical supplies, commodities, finance), and (b) process mechanisms to ensure efficient and effective health service delivery (physical management, procurement, planning, monitoring, information management and governance) (WHO 2000; Knowles et al. 1997). Table 2.1 illustrates a framework of health systems choices, functions, attributes and possible influences on health outcomes.

Similarly, Mills and Ranson (2012, p. 618–619) identified some key actors and key functions appropriate to the health systems (Table 2.2).

Several interrelated aspects need to be considered to have well-functioning, sustainable and affordable health systems that address the wider needs of the people. Lauer et al. (2004, p. 1) argue that health systems should contribute to improving population health, be responsive to the people they serve and be financed fairly assessing against four indicators: 'the level of participation, inequalities in health,

Table 2.1 Functions and impacts of health systems

Health systems choices/ interventions	Process	Intermediate objectives/results	Outcomes
Governance (priority setting, donor coordination, quality standard, health intelligence, public health/health promotion) Financing (resource mobilisation, performance-based payment, subsidised care, evidence-based planning) Generating resources (logistics, manpower, human capital, research and innovation) Organisation of service delivery (decentralization, public-private partnerships, community involvement, quality services) Providing services (personal and population level)	Participation Accountability Representation Resource allocation/ mobilisation Institutional capacity-building	Access Performance Quality Efficiency Equity (utilisation and resource distribution) Choice Accountability Sustainability	Increased use of responsive services Increased use of effective health services—maternal and child health, including reducing the threat of infectious diseases of major health importance Increased use of efficient services

Source: Adapted from PHRplus (2006), p.3; Figueras and McKee (2012)

Table 2.2 Health system actors and their functions

Actors	Key functions
Government and professional body (provides structure and regulates the system) Service users (pay for the health systems to receive health care) Financial institutions (collect/mobilise resources to providers or purchasers) Service providers (level—primary, secondary or tertiary; function—preventive or curative; nature—public or private or a mixed; degree of organisation—formal or informal; types of medical system—allopathic or Ayurvedic services)	• Regulation • Financing • Resource allocation • Provision of services

the level of responsiveness and fairness in financial contribution'. In many parts of the developing world, health systems are too fragile and fragmented to deliver adequate services of sufficient quality (Travis et al. 2004, p. 2). Partners for Health Reformplus (PHRplus 2006, p. 2) further note that despite much effort and resource expenditure on health systems, there is very limited evidence regarding the 'net impact on health-care utilisation and health outcomes'. Similarly, the Centre for Global Development's (2006, p. 2) report also suggests that we need some good evidence from high-quality studies that could appropriately evaluate the effectiveness of health systems and health systems strategies, which might be useful to health sector policy-planners and decision-makers in terms of avoiding 'costly mistakes and prevent doing harm, can identify success, even under adverse circumstances, and can distinguish real successes from apparent successes'. It is, therefore, important to note that strengthening health systems through reforming health services would be considered as an effective approach to developing better health systems.

Activity 1

Which policies and strategies (inputs, processes) are required to bring about positive results (output and outcomes) in health systems development? Give an example related to any health-care intervention from your own country. Discuss.

Health Systems Reform and Decentralization

Health systems, now more than ever before, have not been performing well, and as a result, the level of dissatisfaction is generally high amongst service users, providers, policy-planners and decision-makers. There will be inevitable restructuring or reshaping of existing health services across the world in the light of emerging threats of infectious and chronic diseases of major health importance. Roberts et al. (2004), therefore, strongly advocate the need for a 'health sector reform' movement in health systems. Reform in health relates to positive change, but reform in health systems is not simply any improvement in health services. Sikosana et al. (1997) conceptualise reform in health systems as:

> 'A sustained process of fundamental change in policy and institutional arrangements, guided by government, designed to improve the functioning and performance of the health sector, and ultimately the health status of the population' (p. 3).

As Berman and Bossert (2000, p. 2) note, it is about the 'sustained, purposeful and fundamental change' in health systems, and the key notion of reform is to promise a period of new thinking, thereby bringing innovation in health systems in a way that would be able to address wider health problems. Decentralization is a form of reform mechanism in health systems which usually comes as part of a wider package of public sector health reforms (Wang et al. 2002). Though decentralization has been widely discussed in health sector reform, there is limited agreement in terms of conceptualising its meaning in an appropriate way, as many scholars interpret it differently depending on their own disciplines, motivations and intentions. For example, in the field of public administration, it is more about good governance and less bureaucracy, whilst in the health sector, it is about reshaping the structure and functions of health services for lasting changes in people's health status in the long run (Bankauskaite and Saltman 2007).

Similarly, Oats (1999) argues that there is no clear consensus on which functions and activities should be decentralised, to whom, at what level and in what context, and which are best to keep under central control. In the light of these paradigms, decentralization can be conceptualised as the process of transferring authority and responsibilities with appropriate resources between different scales, usually from central governments to the local authorities. From Hunter et al.'s (1998, p. 310) point of view, it is about a 'shift in power relationships and in the distribution of tasks between levels of government and the various stakeholders to be found at each level'. There are, however, different means and ends of decentralization in general and in health services specifically (see Bossert 1998; Peckham et al. 2005; Saltman et al. 2007) (see Chap. 1 for further details). The key components of health sector reform-related health systems would consist of six key improvements:

- Improving the performance of civil services (restructuring staff, better appraisal systems, performance-related incentives)
- Decentralization (delegating authorities and responsibilities to local governments/agencies)
- Improving the function of health ministries (restructuring, improving human and financial management, stringing policy and planning functions)
- Boarding the health financing options (public-private partnership)
- Introducing managed competition (competition between clinical and support services through single or multiple purchasers)
- Work with the private sector (systems for regulating, contracting or franchising)

Source: Sikosana et al. 1997, p. 4

The World Bank (1993) argues that the primary goal of decentralization is to improve health sector performance and promote social and economic development in the long run. The key notion of decentralization here is that 'smaller organisations, properly structured and steered, are inherently more agile and accountable than larger organisations' (Saltman et al. 2007, p. 1). As Figueras and McKee (2012) argue, decentralization is viewed in many European nations 'as a necessary and local element' of wise stewardship of a health-care system, as Europe contains a large number of geopolitical, economic, legal and organisational variants (p. 235). However, there are several notions of decentralization, concerning whether this can be a panacea to overcome some government challenges in shaping or restructuring public services in the line of people's needs and interests. One common debate amongst scholars is to find an appropriate place for 'decentralization' in 'bureaucratic' governments—we still need more research and investigation in the field of public service reform. Weber

(1947), a German sociologist, first raised the key attributes of the bureaucratic model and concluded that bureaucracy was the fundamental principle of human development, but now he envisaged decentralization as the best alternative to bureaucracy, and his argument was that 'small-scale organisation' would be the best possible option to reach out at people's level (also see Saltman et al. 2007). Health sector reform through decentralization involves some changes and 'sets in different challenges and provides new opportunities for planning, management and development' of health services, including human resources (Wang et al. 2002, p. 441).

It is interesting to note that not all health system changes are health sector reforms. As Berman and Bossert (2000) argue:

> The use of health sector reform in many settings, by many actors with different motivations accounts for some of the negative experiences with health system change. Changes imposed by broad governmental initiates, often with international donor support, usually do not have the explicit goal of improving the health system. Rather, they seek to achieve non-health goals such as macroeconomic stability or more democratic political change. Changes of this type may not produce improvements in health systems or in health (p. 4).

They suggest that on the basis of motive, we can use 'big R', strategic and purposeful, and 'small r', incrementally purposeful, to capture the meaning of reform. In general, 'small r' is considered as a purposeful reform in the health sector. They further argue that:

> Only a few developing countries have undertaken a significant process of health system analysis resulting in planned strategic change. For only a handful of these countries can we observe the impact of such 'big R' reform and draw some conclusion. We should expect that such modest changes would not fundamentally transfer health care systems, although they often result in both positive and negative effects (p. 4).

Activity 2

What should be the overall strategy of decentralization in the health sector? Discuss.

Effective decentralization addresses people's health-care problems through empowering them at the local level, so that they are able to contribute to local health planning and management. As Owino et al. (2000) note, appropriate designs and implementation of decentralization policy would promote access, utilise and coverage to modern health services by the vulnerable people. Owino et al. further argue that this should be part of government's policy framework to promote efficiency and effectiveness in health services delivery. Figueras and McKee (2012, p. 236) clearly highlight that decentralization is such a complex phenomenon that it cannot therefore be a magic bullet for solving 'structure and policy dilemmas', but rather a 'multiple model of configuration' that should fit within the context of national socio- and geopolitical landscapes. It is equally important to bring an important issue; health systems in some areas it are decentralised and other areas are still centrally controlled or recentralised—therefore, as Figueras and McKee (2012) suggest, the key fundamental question remains unanswered about the aspects of health sector decentralization amongst policy-planners and decision-makers, whether 'the mix of decentralization and recentralisation strategies in a given system and the balance between those strategies' would be an appropriate strategy to improve health systems across the world (p. 236).

In addition, WHO (2005) also highlights that weak and inequitable health systems are considered as a key obstacle, including health manpower and sustainable financing to deliver better services across the world. It is therefore important to develop better decentralised systems addressing those challenges to build better and stronger health systems across the world.

Conclusion

Health systems are clearly important to improving health. The global spend on health, US$3.5 trillion, or 8 % of the world's GDP (WHO 2007, p. 9) and the attention given to health systems performance is evidence of this. Many health systems are also undergoing change, often in the context of health sector reforms. When health sector reform efforts have been undertaken, the objective is to improve the performance of the health system so that it is better able to achieve any one or more of the intermediate and/or ultimate goals earlier described. More often than not, the problems that ministries of health confront are interconnected and require a combination of reform strategies. These strategies, in turn, often impact on more than one dimension or level of the health system and on more than one reform goal (Knowles et al. 1997, p. 5).

Health sector reforms typically include decentralization. However, there is only patchy evidence linking improvements in health system performance to decentralization. One problem is that reform can have both intended and unintended consequences, resulting in positive results for one goal but negative effects for another. Empirical studies in Uganda, for instance, determined that following decentralization, local government health planners allocated declining proportions of their budgets to public goods activities (Akin et al. 2005).

Another factor is that the specific technical strategies used to address system performance problems also require broader political, institutional and management actions—such as consensus-building and doing away with bureaucratic constraints—to address the variety of organisational and political obstacles that health sector reform faces (Knowles et al. 1997, p. 6). Further, Newell et al. (2005) observed that a recurring feature in many reform efforts has been a lack of consultation and dialogue to ensure ownership and informed decision-making between those responsible for health systems policy and those tasked with delivering specific interventions.

Health sector reform is a multidimensional process and involves not only defining priorities to be addressed and refining relevant policies but also restructuring the institutions through which health services are delivered. Each country's social and political context is different, and even though some organisational principles are likely to be similar in all reform effort programmes, there is no one-size-fits-all prescription. As Cassels (1995) observed 'the choice of reform options can be influenced by technical advice and analysis, but the decision to proceed, and the subsequent success of implementation, will be dependent on political support'.

To bring lasting change in health systems, and thereby people's health, it is important to capture the wider aspects of population health, financial protection and making services responsive to needs and demands. This means developing sustainable human health manpower, improving functions and structures of governments' health institutions at different levels, strengthening government approaches at local level and improving governance systems at all levels. In addition, secure funding, strong partnerships for health, integrating and coordinating population health services into primary care, local ownership of the services and the level of access and utilisation of essential health-care services are vital attributes of any successful health system.

Further Discussion

- How can the concepts of health sector reform and decentralization be used to assess the performance of a health system? Discuss.
- What are the main areas of health sector reform? Discuss.
- What are the strengths and weaknesses of the health systems in a poor and middle/high income country context?

Recommended Reading

Figueras, J., & McKee, M. (2012). *Health systems, health, wealth and societal well-being*. Maidenhead: Open University Press.

Useful textbook which focuses on health systems from a new perspective. This book also recognises that the roles of health systems include not only improving the health of the population, but also achieving better economic growth.

Johnson, J. A., & Stoskopf, C. H. (2010). *Comparative health systems: Global perspectives for the 21st century*. Sudbury, MA: Jones and Bartlett.

This book compares the health systems of 17 countries using a consistent framework, and explores the global challenges and opportunities for health.

References

Akin, J., Hutchinson, P., & Strumpf, K. (2005). Decentralization and government provision of public goods: The public health sector in Uganda. *The Journal of Development Studies, 41*(8), 1417–1443.

Atun, R. (2012). Health systems, systems thinking and innovation. *Health Policy and Planning, 27*, iv4–iv8.

Bankauskaite, V., & Saltman, R. (2007). Central issues in the decentralization debate. In R. Saltman, V. Bankauskaite, & K. Vrangbaek (Eds.), *Decentralization in healthcare* (pp. 11–27). Maidenhead: Open University Press.

Berman, P. & Bossert, T. (2000) *A decade of health sector reform in developing countries: what have we learned? A Paper prepared for the DDM Symposium – Appraising a decade of health sector reform in developing countries.* Washington DC, March 2000

Bossert, T. (1998). Analysing the decentralization of health systems in developing countries: Decision space, innovation, and performance. *Social Science and Medicine, 47*, 1513–1527.

Busse, R., & Wismar, M. (2002). Health target programmes and health care services—any link? A conceptual and comparative study. *Health Policy, 59*, 209–221.

Cassels, A. (1995). Health sector reform: Key issues in less developed countries. *Journal of International Development, 7*, 329–347.

Centre for Global Development. (2006). *When will we ever learn? Improving lives through impact evaluation. Report of the evaluation working group.* Washington, DC: Centre for Global Development.

Dekker, E. (1994). Healthcare reform and public health. *European Journal of Public Health, 4*, 281–286.

Figueras, J., & McKee, M. (2012). *Health systems, health, wealth and societal well-being.* Maidenhead: Open University Press.

Gilson, L. (1997). *Implementing and evaluating health reform processes: lessons from the literature.* Bethesda, Maryland: Partnerships for Health Reform.

Hafner, T., & Shiffman, J. (2013). The emergence of global attention to health systems strengthening. *Health Policy and Planning, 28*(1), 41–50.

Hunter, D. J., Veinonen, M., & Wlodarczyk, W. C. (1998). Optimal balance of centralised and decentralised management. In R. Saltman, J. Figueras, & C. Sakellarides (Eds.), *Critical challenges in healthcare reform in Europe.* Buckingham: Open University Press.

Knowles, J., Leighton, C., & Stinson, W. (1997). *Measuring health sector reform for system performance: a handbook of indicators.* Bethesda, MD: Partners for Health Reformplus, Abt Associates Inc.

Lauer, J., Lovell, C., Murray, C., & Evans, D. (2004). World health systems performance revisited: the impact of varying the relative importance of health system goals. *BMC Health Services Research, 4*, 19.

Leighton, C. (1996). Strategies for achieving health financing reform in Africa. *World Development, 2*(4), 431–451.

Mills, A., & Ranson, M. (2012). The design of health systems. In M. Merson, R. Black, & A. Mills (Eds.), *Global health: diseases, programs, systems and policies* (pp. 618–619). Burlington, MA: Jones & Bartlett.

Mladovsky, P., Srivastava, D., Cylus, J., Karanikolos, M., Evetovits, T., Thomson, S., & McKee, M. (2012). Health policy in the financial crisis. *EuroHealth: Quarterly of the European Observatory on Health Systems and Policies, 18*(1), 3–6.

Newell, J. N., Collins, C., Baral, S., Omar, M., & Pande, S. (2005). Decentralization and TB control in Nepal: Understanding the views of TB control staff. *Health Policy, 73*(2), 212–227.

Oats, W. E. (1999). An essay on fiscal decentralization. *Journal of Economic Literature, 37*(3), 1120–1149.

Owin, W., Korir, J., Ocholla, P., & Oloo, K. (2000). *Decentralization and health systems development: The question of planning, budgeting and financial structures.* Nairobi, Kenya: Institute of Policy Analysis and Research.

Partners for Health Reformplus. (2006). *Insights for implementation: Improving health systems performance through monitoring and evaluation.* Bethesda, MD: Partners for Health Reformplus, Abt Associates Inc.

Peckham, S., Exworthy, M., Powell, M., & Greener, I. (2005). *Decentralization as an organisational model for healthcare in England.* London: NCCSDO.

Piette, J. D., Lun, K. C., Moura, L. A., Jr., Fraser, H. S., Mechael, P. N., et al. (2012). Impacts of e-health on the outcomes of care in low- and middle-income countries: Where do we go from here? *Bulletin of the World Health Organisation, 90*, 365–372.

Roberts, M., Hsiao, W., Berman, P., & Reich, M. (2004). *Getting health reform right*. Oxford: Oxford University Press.

Roemer, M. I. (1991). *National health systems of the world: Vol 1. The countries*. Oxford: Oxford University Press.

Saltman, R. B. (1994). A conceptual overview of recent healthcare reforms. *European Journal of Public Health, 4*, 287–293.

Saltman, R., Bankauskaite, V., & Vrangbaek, K. (2007). *Decentralization in healthcare*. Maidenhead: Open University Press.

Sikosana, P., Dlamini, Q., & Issakov, A. (1997). *Health sector reform in sub-Saharan Africa: A review of experiences, information gaps and research needs*. Geneva, Switzerland: WHO.

Simon, H. A. (1982). *Models of bounded rationality*. Cambridge, MA: The MIT Press.

Smith, R.D. & Hanson, K. (2011). *Health systems in low- and middle-income countries: An economic and policy perspective*. Oxford Scholarship Online

Thomas, S., Keegan, C., Barry, S., & Layte, R. (2012). The Irish health system and the economic crisis. *The Lancet, 380*(9847), 1056–1057.

Travis, P., Bennett, S., Haines, A., Pang, T., Bhutta, Z., et al. (2004). Overcoming health systems constraints to achieve the Millennium Development Goals. *Lancet, 364*(9437), 900–906.

Wang, Y., Collins, C., Tang, S., & Martineau, T. (2002). Health systems decentralization and human resources management in low and middle income countries. *Public Administration and Development, 22*, 439–453.

Weber, M. (1947). *The theory of social and economic organisation*. New York: Oxford University Press.

World Bank. (1993). *World development report: Investing in health*. New York: Oxford University.

World Health Organization. (2000). *The World Health Report 2000: Health systems: Improving performance*. Geneva, Switzerland: World Health Organization.

World Health Organization. (2005). *Building stronger health systems key to reaching the health Millennium Development Goals*. Geneva, Switzerland: World Health Organization.

World Health Organization. (2006). *Opportunities for global health initiatives in the health system action agenda. Working paper no. 4*. Geneva, Switzerland: World Health Organization.

World Health Organization. (2007). *Everybody's business: Strengthening health systems to improve health outcomes: WHO's framework for action*. Geneva, Switzerland: World Health Organization.

World Health Organization. (2010a). *The World Health Report: Health systems financing: The path to universal coverage*. Geneva, Switzerland: World Health Organization.

World Health Organization. (2010b). *Key components of a well functioning health system*. Geneva, Switzerland: World Health Organization.

Zakus, D., & Bhattacharyya, O. (2007). Health systems, management, and organization in low- and middle-income countries. In W. Markle, M. Fisher, & R. Smego Jr. (Eds.), *Understanding global health*. New York: The McGraw-Hill Companies. http://www.oucom.ohiou.edu/international/updates/UnderstdGlobalHealth_FW_TOC.pdf and http://www.hsph.harvard.edu/takemi/files/2012/10/RP248.pdf (Accessed 17/5/2013).

Chapter 3
Decentralization and Public Health: An Analysis of the Health System in Five Latin American Countries: Argentina, Brazil, Chile, Colombia and Mexico

Gloria Molina, Julian Vargas, and Beatriz Londoño

Abstract This chapter will help you to have an overview of the health sector decentralization process in five Latin American countries, Argentina, Brazil, Chile, Colombia and Mexico, within the context of the wider international health sector reforms introduced in most of the developing countries, during the 1980s and 1990s. The chapter describes the main characteristics of the health systems, the health process and the main socioeconomic and public health indicators of these countries. It also presents a summary of the main findings of several studies focused on analysing the situation of health in these countries. It highlights the fact that decentralization was introduced simultaneously with privatisation, market economy and competition strategies, focalisation and labour flexibility policies, and therefore, it is not easy to conclude if the limitations and achievements of health systems come from it or from the other strategies. Data suggest that with these strategies, problems on accessibility, coverage, quality and inequity of services have not been solved; on the contrary, new barriers of accessibility have been created. The Colombian health system is an example, because the financial profitability interest of the private sector negatively affects efficiency, accessibility and quality, among others.

At the End of the Chapter You Will Be Able to:

- *Identify the main differences and similarities of the health systems and public health indicators between these countries.*
- *Understand the complexity of the decentralizations mixed with privatisation and market economy policies and its implications to accessibility, coverage and quality of health services, especially to the poorest people.*

G. Molina (✉) • J. Vargas • B. Londoño
University of Antioquia, Medellin, Colombia
e-mail: gloria.molina60@gmail.com

K. Regmi (ed.), *Decentralizing Health Services: A Global Perspective*,
DOI 10.1007/978-1-4614-9071-5_3,

Introduction

Decentralization of the health sector has been part of the health sector reforms introduced in the 1980s and 1990s, which have been influenced by international trends, such as:

- Recognition of human rights and a growing awareness that health and human rights are closely related (Legemaate 2002).
- Introduction of the neoliberal economic model (Exworthy and Halford 2002), put in place through the structural adjustment programmes (Granados and Gómez 2000).
- Fiscal crisis and the policies to reduce public expenditure. The financial sustainability was a dominant theme of the health reforms (Islam and Tahir 2002; Bossert 2000).
- Improving capability of the state to undertake and promote collective actions efficiently (The World Bank 1997:3).
- International health policies and agreements: promotion of cost-effective investment in primary care, Alma Ata Conference in 1978, the Ottawa Charter (Griffiths and Crump 1998) and the agreement on healthy cities (WHO 1998), among others.

According to several writers (Islam and Tahir 2002; Mills et al. 2001; Granados and Gómez 2000), health reforms involved strategies such as (a) introducing financial changes such as moving from collective tax-based systems to more individual ones (user charges and compulsory health insurance) and a wide range of resources for health; (b) changing in allocation of resources and paid systems, linking performance and reward; (c) establishing policy priorities for the allocation of public resources for a target population; (d) separation of purchaser and provider, introduction of internal market, contracting out and competition between them; (e) definition of a basic package of services based on cost-benefit criteria; (f) encouraging a wider role to the private sector, both for and not for profit; and (g) transferring policy decision-making, resource management and provision of services from the central to sub-national governments. The main aim of health sector reforms was to improve coverage, quality, accessibility, efficiency and effectiveness of health services.

This chapter is focused on describing and comparing the main characteristics of the decentralization of the health system in five Latin American countries (LAC), Argentina, Brazil, Chile, Colombia and Mexico, in which health sector reforms were introduced at the end of the 1980s and at the beginning of the 1990s. It also includes the main public health indicators and some findings of the process coming from several studies carried out in the 1990s and 2000s, which were focused on analysing the achievements in relation to efficiency, quality and accessibility of health services.

Decentralization of the Health Sector

Decentralization is a complex public policy that involves fiscal, institutional, administrative, social and political issues; it entails transferring resources, decision-making, planning and management functions from the central government to subordinate units of the government, semi-autonomous public corporations, local government, regional organisations and/or specialised authorities. It includes expanding formal authority from a smaller to a larger number of actors (Rondinelli 1990:9; López 1995:4). It is closely associated with democracy because it involves citizen participation (Rondinelli 1990), political development of society, distribution of power, changes of the role and legitimacy of the state (Pollitt et al. 1998). It is grounded on the principal-agent approach, which means that a principal (e.g. Ministry of Health) is entrusting funds to an agent (e.g. sub-national level or hospital) with the intention that some desired health-care delivery can be secured. The principal-agent relationship implies the existence of a contract (either explicit or implicit) under which one or more persons/institutions (the principal) engage another person or persons/institutions (as agent) to perform a service on their behalf (Smith et al. 1997:38, 41).

Some researchers agree with the following classification of decentralization: de-concentration, delegation, devolution and privatisation (Rondinelli 1990; Mills et al. 1990). However, in practice, there have been mixtures of them. Privatisation allows services to be provided by several types of institutions and organisations that include community groups, cooperatives and individuals. But there has been controversy because seeing privatisation as a model of decentralization has generated confusion and, in some cases, rejection because of the effects of market failures (Collins and Green 1993:59). Rojas (1999) suggests that almost all LAC have adopted a reform of the state and/or of some public services such as health and education, the election of mayors rather than their being appointed. According to Castañeda et al. (1999) and Londoño et al. (1999), the main functions transferred from the central to sub-national government levels in most LAC are as follows: (a) financial issues; (b) human resources (hiring, firing and contract process); (c) supplies and investment decisions; (d) planning, surveillance and control; (e) health service organisation; (f) access rules; and (g) governance rules (facility boards, district offices and community participation).

Public Health

According to Rothstein (2002) and Franco (1993), public health is concerned with community health as a whole; public health is community health. The mission of public health is to fulfil society's interest in assuring conditions under which people can be healthy. The public health core functions could be summarised as follows: (a) to promote health as human right; (b) to formulate and put in place public health policies based on local, regional and national health problems and priorities; (c) to ensure that all populations have access to appropriate and cost-effective care; and

(d) assessing and monitoring of health in communities and populations at risk by identifying health problems and priorities.

Public health is also related to constitutional human rights and duties and social, economic, cultural and institutional public policies; to the development model, incomes, employment, housing, education, meanings and practices of health; and to the roles of the state, the private sector and the community. In this sense, the OMS (2008) recognises that the social determinants of health are the conditions in which people are born, grow, live and work. These circumstances are shaped by the distribution of money, power and resources at global, national and local levels. The social determinants of health are mostly responsible for health inequities—the unfair and avoidable differences in health status seen within and between countries (OMS 2008). In this context, primary health care (PHC) is a strategy to improve health and human development of the population, because it involves an intersectoral network to tackle different problems that affect health (OPS 2007). In this sense, decentralization should allow us the implementation of PHC strategy at the municipal and regional levels.

Public health actions such as prevention and monitoring of transmissible diseases, quality of water supply, sewerage, quality of air and environmental contamination, among others, are considered public goods and services (Scott 2001:26–7; Batley 1996:728) due to their characteristics of having no rival and no exclusion (Yadón et al. 2006:12) and also their externalities. In the decentralization of the health sector, municipal and regional authorities are accountable for the provision of public goods and services such as public health programmes according to population needs, because they are closer to the community needs. Therefore, it is expected that the decentralization of the health sector generates (a) more efficiency in providing services according to the needs of the local population; (b) innovation and adaptation of services according to the local conditions; (c) better accessibility and quality of services, transparency, accountability and legitimacy related to more community participation in decision-making and surveillance processes; and (d) more equity in the distribution of resources among regions (Banco Mundial 1998).

Main Demographic and Social Indicators of the Five Countries

Table 3.1 shows the data of some demographic and social indicators for each country. Brazil has the largest population, followed by Mexico and Colombia; Argentina and Chile have the smallest population of the five countries. Fertility rate is very similar in the five countries, between 1.9 children per woman, the lowest in Chile and the highest in Mexico. Brazil shows the lowest birth rate with 16.1 and Argentina the highest with 18.9 per 1,000 population. Life expectancy is around 73 years old in Brazil and 78 years old in Chile. The population under the poverty line is different among the five countries. Colombia has the highest percentage with 45.5 % of the population under the poverty line and Argentina has the lowest with 13.9 %. The five countries involve different forms and scope of social security insurance in health, and it is difficult to compare them. Colombia exhibits the highest percentage of population with health insurance (88.7 %), because the whole health system is based

Table 3.1 Main demographic and social indicators of five Latin American countries

Indicators	Argentina (2008)	Brazil	Chile	Colombia	México
Total population	40.518.951[a]	189.953.000[b]	17.094.270[c]	45.509.584[d]	112.336.538[e]
Fertility rate	2.3[f]	2.3(2008)[b]	1.9[c]	2.2[g]	2.4[e]
Birth rate	18.9(2009)[f]	16.1(2008)[h]	15.0(2009)[i]	17.7[g]	17.8[e]
Life expectancy	75.2 years[a]	73 years	78 years[c]	75[d]	75.4[e]
Percentage of population under the poverty line	13.9[j]	26(2008)[j]	15.1[c]	45.5(2009)[g]	18.2[j]
Population covered by social security	44.9[a]	–	16.9[i]	88.7[k]	43.0[e]
Population not covered by social security	53.03[a]	–	5.1(2006)[i]	11.1[k]	27.7[e]
Total expenditure on health as percentage GDP	9.6[a]	9.0[j]	8.4 (2009)[l]	6.4(2009)[g]	5.9[e]
Total expenditure on health per capita	1 385[a]	645.27 public[m] 837.35 private	1 186 (2009)[l]	472 (2007–2010)[n]	890[e]

[a] Bell, M., Becerril-Montekio, V. M. (2011). Sistema de salud de Argentina. *Salud Pública Méx.* 53(suppl 2), S96-S108

[b] Instituto brasileiro de Geografia y Estatistica (IBGE). (2008). Aspectos Demográficos. http://www.ibge.gov.br/home/estatistica/populacao/condicaodevida/indicadoresminimos/tabela1.shtm. Accessed 18 jul 2012

[c] Gobierno de Chile, Departamento de Estadísticas e Información de Salud (DEIS), Ministerio de Salud. (s. f.). *Indicadores básicos en salud 2010.* Chile: Autor. http://deis.minsal.cl/. Accessed 18 jul 2012

[d] Departamento Nacional de Estadística (DANE). *Proyecciones de Población.* Bogotá: Autor. http://www.dane.gov.co/index.php?option=com_content&view=article&id=75&Itemid=72. Accessed 21 jul 2012

[e] Instituto Nacional de Estadística y Geografía (INEGI) (s. f.). *Información Nacional, por entidad federativa y municipios.* México: Autor. http://www.inegi.org.mx/sistemas/mexicocifras/default.aspx. Accessed 21 jul 2012

[f] Instituto Nacional de Estadística y Censos (INDEC). *Dirección Nacional de Estadísticas Sociales y de Población. Estimaciones y proyecciones de población total país 1950–2015.* Buenos Aires: Autor. http://www.indec.mecon.ar/. Accessed 21 jul 2012

[g] INDEXMUNDI (s. f). *Tasa de natalidad.* http://www.indexmundi.com/g/g.aspx?v=25&c=co&l=es. Accessed 21 jul 2012

[h] WIKIPEDIA (s. f.). *Demografía de Brasil.* http://es.wikipedia.org/wiki/Demograf%C3%ADa_de_ Brasil#Indicadores_b.C3.A1sicos. Accessed 30 jul 2012

[i] Gobierno de Chile, Departamento de Estadísticas e Información de Salud (DEIS), Ministerio de Salud. (2009). *Estadísticas de Natalidad y Mortalidad Chile, Año 2009.* Chile: Autor. http://deis.minsal.cl/vitales/anuarios/2009/Anuario_2009_vitales.pdf. Accessed 30 jul 2012

[j] INDEXMUNDI (s. f). *Población bajo el nivel de pobreza (%).* http://www.indexmundi.com/g/g.aspx?v=69&c=ar&l=es. Accessed 19 jul 2012

[k] Departamento Nacional de Estadística (DANE) (2012). *Encuesta nacional de calidad de vida 2011.* Bogotá: Autora. http://www.dane.gov.co/files/investigaciones/condiciones_vida/calidad_vida/Boletin_Prensa_ECV_2011.pdf. Accessed 19 jul 2012

[l] Gobierno de Chile, Ministerio de Salud. *Panorama de salud 2011 informe sobre Chile y comparación con países miembros.* Chile: Autor. http://www.eligevivirsano.cl/wp-content/uploads/2012/01/Panorama-de-la-Salud-2011.pdf. Accessed 21 jul 2012

[m] Instituto brasileiro de Geografía y Estadística (IBGE) (2012). *Cuenta Satélite de Salud Brasil - 2007–2009 Consumo de bienes y servicios de salud llega al 8,8 % del PIB.* Brasil: Autor. http://www.ibge.gov.br/espanhol/presidencia/noticias/noticia_impressao.php?id_noticia=2070. Accessed 26 July 2012

[n] Banco Mundial. (s. f.). *Gasto en salud per cápita (US$ a precios actuales).* Washington D. C.: Autor. http://datos.bancomundial.org/indicador/SH.XPD.PCAP. Accessed 26 jul 2012

Sources: See list of references at the end of the chapter

on insurance as a way to get access to services; the Brazilian health system is funded by general taxes; the other countries have different approaches of insurance.

The total health expenditure as percentage of the GDP is similar in the five countries: Mexico has the lowest figure with 5.9 % and Argentina has the highest with 9.6 %. In the per capita health expenditure, there are also important differences among these five countries: Argentina has the highest with US $ 1.385 and Colombia has the lowest with US$ 472.

General Characteristics of the Decentralization and the Health System in Each Country

Argentina

In Argentina the health decentralization process began with the Provincial Constitution of 1987 (Ase 2006); the provinces are responsible for the health care and protection of its population. In the 1990s, decentralization of health services looked for improving accessibility, efficiency and quality of care and strengthened promotion and protection of target vulnerable groups. The Ministry of Health (MOH) was freed from the direct management of services and transferred funds to the provinces, gaining budgetary availability to finance priority programmes. Social security and the public sector rose from supply subsidies to demand subsidies. Free choice of participants and competition among them was implemented through deregulation in Obras Sociales (OS) and prepaid medical companies (EMP). Then, the Ministry of Health and Welfare, MSAS (Decree No. 486 of February 2002) was reformed in order to improve coordination with the provinces (PAHO 2001:6). The municipalities with greater economic power and larger population manage their own resources and have the authority to schedule and conduct health actions independently.

Main Characteristics of the Health System in Argentina

Stewardship, Monitoring and Control
The Ministry of Health and Social Assistance (MSAS) has various decentralised agencies: the Superintendency of Health Services (SSS) with administrative, economic and financial autonomy; some non-decentralised hospitals; and the Institute for Retirees and Pensioners (PAMI). The primary role of the MSAS is intersectoral negotiation, the establishment of policies and standards, monitoring and dissemination of information. The Federal Health Council (COFESA), composed of the Minister of Health and the Secretaries of the provinces and the city of Buenos Aires, is the space of building institutional consensus, goal setting, policymaking and shared decisions between

(continued)

sectors and jurisdictions. The SSS monitors compliance with the Compulsory Medical Plan (PMO) and the implementation of the National Quality Assurance in Medical Care (PNGCAM), monitors compliance with the free choice of the Obras Sociales (OS) by the beneficiaries and convenes annual public hearings to discuss health issues of concern to the public. The MSAS has the National Epidemiological Surveillance System, whose data are mostly in the public sector (MSAS 1994).

Financing and Service Delivery
The health sector includes three subsectors: (a) the public sector composed of provincial and national administrative structures responsible for conducting a sector and the public hospital network. It is funded with fiscal resources and receives occasional payments from the social security system; (b) the compulsory social insurance subsector organised by Obras Sociales (OS), nearly 300, is financed by contributions from workers and employers. Each province has an OS that covers public employees under their jurisdiction; (c) the private subsector comprising independent professionals, hospitals and private clinics that serve individual users and beneficiaries of the OS, using different methods of payment. It also includes the prepaid medical enterprises (EMP). The OS covered between 1998 and 2008 a population of about 18.3 million people (45 %) (Belló and Becerril 2011:5). Most of them provide services in their institutions and through contracts with private providers (Superintendencia de Servicios de Salud Argentina 2010). The national OS and EMP provide a Compulsory Medical Plan (PMO) including facilities and medicines. Public hospitals provide services to the population on demand and act as a reassurance to the OS. The MSAS, provinces and some large municipalities develop vertical public health programmes to the targeted population and also environmental programmes (PAHO/WHO 1997).

Brazil

In Brazil, the Ministry of Welfare and Social Assistance was created in 1974; the project for integrated health started in 1983. In 1988 the new Constitution created the Unified Health System (SUS), which was regulated in 1990 by the Health Law. In 1997 came the creation of basic care and there were transfers per capita from the federal level to municipalities (Becerril et al. 2011a, b:4). In 2006, the Covenant Health priority areas of the SUS, regionalisation processes, investment, planning and scheduling tools were defined. The National Regulatory Policy was structured and implemented (Guimarães 2004:303–327; CONASS 2003). The 2004–2007 Plan aimed for social inclusion and reduction of social inequalities.

During the government of Lula da Silva (2008–2011), the programme "Better Health: A Right for Everyone" included among its strategies the following: universal health system, equitable and comprehensive actions associated with economic and social development; health promotion, social participation and intersectoral approach; prioritising the objectives of the Pact for health; deepening regionalisation and federalism; and raising the quality and efficiency of the units producing goods and health services (ABRASCO et al. 2010; Aquino et al. 2009).

Main Characteristics of the Health System in Brazil

Stewardship, Monitoring and Control

In the Unified Health System (SUS) of Brazil, the service network at each level of government is under the leadership of the Ministry of Health (MOH), the State Secretariats of Health (SES) and the Municipal Health Department (MHD). National, State and Municipal Health Councils, with government representatives, professionals, providers and users, set guidelines and targets in each territory, under the recommendations of health conferences, which are defined at the three spheres of government, in which there is broad participation of society through calls quadrennial Executive Branch (OPS 2005:15). The MOH, the national council and federal agencies are involved in funding, coordinating, monitoring and evaluating the system; they also define technical standards and coordinate health and epidemiological surveillance and health information systems.

In 1998, the Health National Surveillance System was created, and a set of institutions coordinated by the National Health Surveillance Agency (Bahia 2005:9–30). The MOH exerts its control through five departments: Executive, Health Care, Science, Technology and Strategic Inputs, Labour Management and Health Education and Participatory Management. The SUS Management Pact established the municipal and state monitoring and evaluation of services and the definition of indicators to perform the monitoring (Teixeira and Costa 2008: 795–817). Since 2006, it operates a set of planning and scheduling tools, goals and commitments to public health actions that involve federal, state and municipal levels (Galilea et al. 2011).

The system has four objectives: (a) universal care without restrictions, (b) equity, (c) integrity of the individual and collective actions and (d) environmental care (Becerril et al. 2011a, b:9).

Financing and Service Delivery

The SUS is financed through taxes and social contributions at the three levels of government: federal, state and municipal levels. Health, social security and social assistance are financed from the budget of the union, states, federal district and municipalities, with social contributions from employers

(continued)

and workers, and taxes on gambling (OPS 2005:1). The constitutional reform of 2000 defined the sources of resources for health (Ugá and Porto 2008). In 2008 the Senate passed a new regulation, and in 2011, the federation earmarked at least 10 % of their income for health, the states and the federal district 12 % and 15 % from the municipalities (Barros 2003; OPS 2005). Budgets of SUS are deposited on the health funds (Bermudez et al. 2008:435–472).

The health system combines three approaches: (a) the public one covering 75 % of the population and the private one the remaining 25 %. SUS services are decentralised through a network of clinics and hospitals; (b) the private network is concentrated in the most industrialised and economically developed areas of the country and is subjected to regulation, supervision and control of the state (CF art 197–199). Part of the population covered by the private system also uses the public network for complex and costly procedures; (c) the Family Health Programme seeks universal coverage, grounded in primary health-care approach, through health teams serving both health units and at home. The minimum equipment consists of doctors, nurses, nursing assistants and community health leaders. In 2002, 65 % of hospitals were private, while 76 % of outpatient facilities were public (OPS 2005:14).

Chile

Health sector decentralization in Chile started in the 1980s, when the primary care provision was transferred to the municipalities; therefore, the municipality was responsible for most urban and rural general practices, rural health posts and rural medical centres. Resources, planning, management and decision-making were transferred to providers of services. The authority to appoint and dismiss staff that had been decentralised was re-centralised, and nowadays, all the staff belongs to the national civil service (Rivas s.f). With decentralization, the Municipal Common Fund was created, redistributing a portion of the resources of the richer municipalities to poorer ones in order to improve equity (Bossert 2000:9). The implementation of decentralization has gone through several stages during the 1980s and was fully implemented upon the restoration of democracy in 1989; it was implemented simultaneously with the reform of the social security system, which encouraged the creation of private health plans through the Instituciones de Salud Previsional (ISAPRE) and an expansion of private provision. After 1989, the democratic government allocated more resources to public health (Bossert 2000:9).

Health services are organised in 29 Regional Health Services consisting of hospitals, general urban and rural medical rooms, rural health posts and rural health medical centre that provide inpatient and outpatient services for members of the FONASA. Also, they carry out actions to promote and protect recovery and rehabilitation of health (Becerril et al. 2011:136).

Main Characteristics of the Health System in Chile

Stewardship, Monitoring and Control
The National Public Health Service (NPHS) in Chile is composed of the Ministry of Health (MOH) and its regional and municipal institutions, the Public Health Institute (PHI), the National Supply Central (CENABAST), the National Fund for Health Service (FONASA) and the Superintendency of Health (Vergara and Martinez 2006: 512; Becerril et al. 2011:133). The MOH leads the system, develops policies, plans and programmes, sets standards and assesses and monitors the performance of the institutions that comprise it. It also regulates and supervises the first-level care provided by the Municipal System in Health Care. There is a Department of Health as part of the municipal authority, under the supervision of the MOH. The PHI is responsible for public health, supervising and evaluating the quality of laboratories, conducting disease surveillance and monitoring the drugs produced and sold in Chile, the environmental and occupational health and production and quality control of vaccines. CENABAST buys and distributes medicines, supplies and medical equipment for the NHS. The Superintendency of Health monitors and controls the ISAPRE, FONASA, the Health Guarantees Regime and the public and private health providers. The Department of Statistics and Health Information collects, consolidates and validates data, in order to set health policies (Becerril et al. 2011:139–140; Reyes and Annick 2011).

Financing and Service Delivery
Resources to finance the health system come from general taxation, mandatory contributions of employers and employees, contributions to private voluntary health insurance, pocket spending and donations. There are two types of insurance:

1. The National Health Fund (FONASA) collects, manages and distributes health funds, which come from taxes and mandatory health premiums for workers who choose it as insurance. It covers 70 % of the population, especially the rural and urban poor, lower middle class and retirees (Becerril et al. 2011:132). FONASA offers two models of health care: a) Institutional Care Model in public institutions, where the beneficiaries pay for care based on their income and people with the lowest income do not pay, and b) Free Choice Model (MLE) in private providers, for people with the highest income. FONASA has a central structure, decentralised territorially (Vergara and Martinez 2006: 512–513).
2. The Instituciones de Salud Previsional (ISAPRE) are private insurers that manage the compulsory contributions of workers who choose them. They cover 17.5 % of the population, those with the highest incomes, and provide services in their own facilities, also in the public and private health institutions.

(continued)

In 2005 the following new laws were introduced: Health Authority and Management Law, which separates the service delivery functions of regulation, strengthens the health authority and creates a system of accreditation of public and private institutions; the General Law on Health Fair, which led to the Universal Access Plan with Explicit Guarantees for 56 diseases, including those of high cost; The Solvency Act of ISAPRE, which ensures stability of system and protects members in situations of insolvency; and Amendment Act which ensures ISAPRE's operation, improving transparency and enhancing the role of the Superintendence of Health (Becerril et al. 2011:141).

Colombia

Decentralization of the health sector in Colombia started with Law 12 of 1986 and Decree 77 of 1987, which led to decentralised investment in infrastructure of primary health care, and assigned responsibilities for building and maintenance of the health centres, hospitals and the provision of water and basic sanitation. With the election of mayors and governors, the process moved from delegation and de-concentration towards devolution. Law 10 of 1990 involved a territorial and institutional decentralization, allocating responsibility for the managing health services to 1,009 mayors and 32 governors elected in 1988; it also increased fiscal resources for health. Then, the National Constitution of 1991 emphasised political decentralization and transferred decision-making power, which meant more resources and responsibilities from national to sub-national levels (Sarmiento 2004:9). These constitutional mandates were put in place through Law 60 and Law 100 of 1993; the last one created the Social Security System for Health (SSSH) based on decentralization, solidarity, equity, universality, integrity, unity, efficiency, effectiveness and participation. It also introduced privatisation, competition and market mechanisms and allocated new functions on the regional and municipal governments related to managing the subsidised scheme, surveillance and control of the institutions delivering health services.

Main Characteristics of the Colombian Health System

Stewardship, Monitoring and Control

The current structure of the Colombian health system is composed mainly of the Ministry of Health (MOH), the Regional/Departmental and Municipal Health Directorates, the Superintendency of Health, The National Institute of

(continued)

Health, the private and public health insurers (Health Promoter Enterprises: Empresas Promotoras de Salud, EPS) and providers (Instituciones Prestadoras de Servicios de Salud, IPS) and the Solidarity and Guarantee Fund (FOSYGA). The Ministry of Health (MOH) leads the system and establishes policies and general legislation. With decentralization, MOH no longer operates hospitals; the Departmental Health Directorate is responsible for the health sector and the public hospitals of second level of complexity. Municipal Health Directorate and mayors are responsible for the municipal public hospitals and health centres to provide primary health care. Mayors became the political and managerial leaders of the health sector and coordinators of multi-sector activities in their municipalities. The National Superintendency of Health must accomplish surveillance and control functions of the whole system throughout the country, with the cooperation of the MOH and the Departmental and Municipal Health Authorities. The EPS manages the subsidy and contributory scheme. Act 715 of 2001 created the general system of fiscal resources; the central level retained the role of planner and policymaker, coordinator and monitor of the municipalities on the health matters (Law 10 of 1990; Law 60 of 1993; Law 100 of 1993).

Financing and Provision of Services

The Colombian health system has a mixed financing, which is managed by the Solidarity and Guarantee Fund (FOSYGA). Its resources come from compulsory contributions by 12.5 % of the monthly salary (8.5 % of the employers and 4 % of the employees) to the contributory scheme; compulsory insurance to traffic accident—SOAT (Spanish initials), weapon taxes, Cajas de Compensación, National Budget Counterpart and petroleum/oil revenues, among others (Law 100, 1993). There are also Municipal Participations of the National Revenues allocated as follows: 30 % for education; 25 % for health (to subsidy scheme and to the poor population's non-affiliates to the social security system and to public health programmes); 20 % for water and basic sanitary services; 5 % for sports, recreation and cultural activities; and 20 % for free investment in public services (Law 60 of 1993, Art. 10 and 22).

Health services are provided by public and private institutions (IPS). Since 1993, the number of private providers has increased significantly, especially those of high technology and cost services that generate high profitability. At the same time, the provision of primary health-care services and especially public health programmes has decreased because these services are not profitable to private providers. Public hospitals became autonomous (Empresas Sociales del Estado) and compete with private ones for the provision of services, through contracting out process with private and public insurers, Departmental and Municipal Health Directorate. Public health programmes to the poorest people are provided mainly by the public hospitals paid by the municipal government.

Mexico

In 1979 and 1988, Mexico introduced structural, legislative and administrative changes within the health services for the population not affiliated to social security. In 1983 the right to health protection was included in the Constitution; then the General Act of 1984 and state health laws were issued. The first strategies were institutional sectoring, modernisation of the Ministry of Health and Welfare, intersectoral coordination, community participation and decentralization of health services, which took place in two stages: the first one in 1983 in 14 states and the second one in 1993 in the remaining states and the capital district. Other strategies for human resource development in health, health information, funding and supplies for the National Health Services were introduced. This reform emphasised primary health care. In 1995 the decentralization of the MOH extended to all the states, a basic package of 13 health interventions for the dispersed rural population was defined, hospitals and medical schools were certified, the Medical Arbitration Commission was created and the insurance institutions specialising in health were regulated. The emphasis of this reform was on replacing the vertical and segmented model with a new universal, participatory and pluralistic one. It also created the Program of Action in Field Performance Assessment 2001–2006 to assess the achievements of decentralization (Jaramillo 2007b: 87–88).

Characteristics of the Health System in Mexico

Stewardship, Monitoring and Control

The health system in Mexico is composed of two sectors: public and private. The public sector includes social security institutions (the Mexican Social Security Institute (IMSS), the Institute of Security and Social Services for State Workers (ISSSTE), Petroleos Mexicanos (PEMEX), the Secretary of National Defense (SEDENA) and the Secretary of the Navy (SEMAR)) that provide services to workers in the formal sector of the economy; the institutions that protect and serve the population without social security are the Popular Health Insurance (SPS-Seguro Popular de Salud), the Secretariat of Health (SSa), the State Health Services (SESA) and IMSS-Opportunities Program (IMSS-O). The private sector provides services to people with the ability to pay (Gómez-Dantés et al. 2011:221).

The health system in Mexico has gone through several reforms in order to achieve greater efficiency and effectiveness in the delivery of health services. The government, during 2000–2006, introduced in 2003 the Social Protection System in Health, known as Seguro Popular de Salud (SPS), for the population not covered by social security. The SPS transfers the federal funds based on the number of families who enrol in the programme and therefore represents a

(continued)

recentralisation of decision-making (Homedes and Ugalde 2011:494; Jaramillo 2007a:87–88). According to FUNSALUD (2012:24), in spite of reforms, the Mexican health system still needs to overcome current problems such as inequity, financial insecurity, poor quality, inadequate information, inertia and vested interests.

Financing and Provision of Services
The financing of social security institutions comes from three sources: government contributions, employer contributions (in the case of ISSSTE, PEMEX, SEMAR SEDENA and the government are the same) and employee contributions. These institutions provide services in their own hospitals and with their own staff. The SSA and the SESA are funded by the federal government and state governments, and recovery fees are paid by users. They also offer services to people in their own facilities. The SPS is funded by the federal government, state governments and family fees; it buys health services to SSA, the SESA and in some cases to private entities. Finally, the private sector is financed by payments made by users when receiving care and private health insurance premiums and provides services in private hospitals (Gómez-Dantés et al. 2011:221).

Main Public Health Indicators of the Five Countries

Vaccination is one of the most important public health programmes, especially for children, against transmissible diseases. The Expanded Programme on Immunisation (EPI) was established in 1974 through a World Health Assembly resolution (resolution WHA27.57) focused on the global smallpox eradication programme and to ensure that all children in all countries benefited from life-saving vaccines. Table 3.2 shows the percentage of children vaccinated with DPT, tuberculosis and measles. Argentina had low percentage of coverage with DPT in 1990–2000, but increased in 2005–2010; with the other vaccines, it achieved a coverage of over of 93 %. Brazil had low coverage of vaccination with DPT and measles in 1990–1995, but it improved from 2000 to 2010, achieving a coverage of 95–100 % of the children. Chile has had a coverage of over 90 %, but the coverage with DPT and measles decreased in 2000–2010. Colombia shows ups and downs from 1990 to 2010 in the coverage with the three vaccines; it draws attention on the decrease of coverage of DPT in 2000, of measles in 1995–2000 and of TB in 2000–2010, during the implementation of the Health Social Security System. Finally, Mexico had low coverage in 1990, but it increased progressively, getting coverage of 95–100 %. The indicators on coverage of vaccination are similar in Colombia and Chile, where the health systems are dominated by the competitive market and private insurers.

Table 3.2 Percentage of vaccination coverage in five Latin American countries (1990, 1995, 2000, 2005, 2010)

	DPT					Tuberculosis-TB					Measles				
Countries	1990[a]	1995[b]	2000[a]	2005	2010	1990	1995	2000	2005	2010	1990	1995	2000	2005	2010
Argentina	87	85	83	94	95	100	100	100	100	100	93	99	91	100	100
Brazil	66	81	98	96	96	79	100	100	100	100	78	87	99[a]	100	98
Chile	95	94	91	91	92	94	97	93	95	96	97	97	97	90	93
Colombia	88	94	79	93	88	95	100	91	94	84	82	61	80	94	89
Mexico	53	91	97	98	95	67	98	100	99	98	75	90	96	96	95

[a]Organización Mundial de la Salud (OMS) (2010). *Estadísticas sanitarias Mundiales 2010*. Ginebra: Autor. http://www.who.int/gho/publications/world_health_statistics/ES_WHS10_Full.pdf. Accessed 23 jul 2012

[b]Pan American Health Organization (PAHO) (2010). *Coverage in the Americas by Country.* http://ais.paho.org/phip/viz/im_coveragebycountry.asp. consultado 26 de julio de 2012. Accessed 26 jul 2012

Source: See list of references at the end of the chapter

Table 3.3 Tuberculosis mortality rate per 100.000 inhabitants in five Latin American countries (2000–2009[a])

Country	2000	2005	2009
Argentina	2.2	1.7	1.4
Brazil	3.1	2.5	2.5
Chile	1.8	1.4	1.4
Colombia	3.0	2.6	2.3 (2008)
Mexico	3.2	2.3	1.9

[a]Pan American Health Organization (PAHO) (s.f.). *Regional Mortality Information System. Corrected mortality rates. 2011*. http://www.paho.org/Spanish/SHA/coredata/tabulator/newsqlTabulador.asp. Accessed 23 jul 2012

Source: See list of references at the end of the chapter

Tuberculosis is one of the transmissible diseases linked to the social and economic conditions of the population. It is also an indicator of the capacity of the health system to prevent it by carrying out strategies for timely diagnosis and provision of the treatment. Table 3.3 shows that Argentina and Chile have the lowest mortality rate by tuberculosis, while Brazil, Colombia and Mexico have the highest mortality rate, which is coherent with the percentage of population under poverty line presented above.

Table 3.4 exhibits data on general, infant and maternal mortality rates of the five countries: Argentina, Brazil, Chile, Colombia and Mexico. The five countries show a progressive decrease of the general and infant mortality rate from 1990 to 2010. Maternal mortality rate decreased from 1990 to 2000, but in 2005 and 2010, it increased in Argentina, Brazil, Chile and Colombia. Mexico exhibited a progressive decrease of maternal mortality rate from 1990 to 2010. In 2010, Argentina had the highest general mortality rate (7.4, 7.7) and Mexico had the lowest (4.7); Brazil had the highest infant mortality rate (21.9) and Chile had the lowest (7.5); Colombia exhibits the highest maternal mortality rate (72.9) and Chile the lowest (19.7). Among the five countries, Chile has the lowest general, infant and maternal mortality rates and also in other social and economic indicators presented in Table 3.1, such as life expectancy.

Low quality and disintegration of the health information systems are one of the problems identified in these countries, which could be the explanation of different figures of mortality rate for the same period in some countries. It seems that the information system is not unified. It stands in the Colombian case due to failures of the information system among several actors: insurers, providers and governmental entities (Table 3.4).

The profile of morbidity and mortality of a population is related to the social determinants of health (OMS 2008) and the capacity of a health system to promote health and provide high-quality services to prevent risks and give treatment and rehabilitation to patients. Table 3.5 shows that the mortality profile has changed during the last 15 years in the five countries. While in the 1990s the infectious diseases were within the five main general causes of death, in 2007–2010 the chronic

Table 3.4 General, infant and maternal mortality rate of five Latin American countries (1990–2010)

	General mortality rate per 1,000 people				
Countries	1990	1995	2000	2005	2010
Argentina	8.0[a]	7.7[a] 7.9[b]	7.5[a] 7.8[b] 7.59[c]	7.6[a] 7.56[c]	7.39[c] 7.7[b]
Brazil	–	6.6[b]	9.37[c] 6.4[b] 6.63[k]	6.15[c]	6.35[c] 6.4[b]
Chile	–	5.4[b]	5.52[c] 5.1[b]	5.76[b]	5.9[c] 5.6[b]
Colombia	–	6.21[d] 6.0[b]	5.73[c] 5.95[d]	5.59[c] 5.81[d]	5.24[c] 5.80[d]
Mexico	5.6[e]	5.0[e]	5.05[c] 4.8[b] 4.9[e]	4.73[c] 4.8[e]	4.83[c] 4.7[b] 5.0[e]
	Infant mortality rate per 1,000 live births				
Countries	1990	1995	2000	2005	2010
Argentina	24[f]	22.2[a]	16.6[a] 18.31[c]	8.9[a] 15.18[c]	8.0[a] 11.11[c]
Brazil	46[f]	–	38.04[c] 27.4[g] 30.1 (see table footnote j of Table 1)	29.61[c] 21.4[c]	21.86[c]
Chile	18[f]	–	9.6[c]	8.8[c]	7.52[c]
Colombia	41.40[h] 28[f]	28.40[d] 35.20[h]	20.41[i] 24.7[c] 25.6[h]	15.91[i] 20.97[c] 22.00[h] 22.25[d]	13.89[i] 16.87[c] 19.10[h]
Mexico	39.2[e]	27.6[e]	26.19[c] 19.4[e]	20.91[c] 16.76[e]	17.84[c] 14.2[e]
	Maternal mortality rate per 100,000 live births				
Countries	1990	1995	2000	2005	2009–2010
Argentina	80.0[a]	44.0[a]	35.0[j]	39.0[a]	55.0[a] 40 (2008) (see table footnote a of Table 1)
Brazil	143.2[g]	115.7[c]	73.2[g] 45.8[k]	74.7[c]	–
Chile	56[f]	–	18.7[l]	19.7[l]	19.7[l]
Colombia	88.0[m] 87.0[n]	61.0[m] 63[n]	104.94[o] 101.7[m] 105[n]	73.06[f] 70.1[m]	62.76 (2008)[n] 72.88[o]
Mexico	89.0[a,p]	83.2[a]	72.6[a]	61.8[a]	51.5[a]

[a] Instituto Nacional de Estadística y Censos de la República. *Síntersis de coyuntura.* Argentina: Autor. http://www.indec.mecon.ar/. Accessed 21 jul 2012

[b] Pan American Health Organization (PAHO) (s. f.). *Health Indicators database, 2009.* Washington D.C.: Autor. Recuperado el 22 de Julio de 2012 en http://ais.paho.org/phip/viz/basicindicatorbrowaser.asp

(continued)

Table 3.4 (continued)

[c] INDEXMUNDI (s. f). *Tasa de mortalidad (muertes/1000 habitantes).* http://www.indexmundi.com/g/g.aspx?v=26&c=co&l=es. Accessed 21 jul 2012

[d] DANE Departamento Nacional de Estadística. (s. f.) *Proyecciones de población 2006–2020.* Bogotá: Autor. http://www.dane.gov.co/index.php?option=com_content&view=article&id=73&Itemid=119. Accessed 19 jul 2012

[e] Concejo Nacional de Población (CONAPO) (s. f.). *Indicadores demográficos básicos 1990–2030.* México: Autor. http://www.conapo.gob.mx/es/CONAPO/Indicadores_demograficos_basicos. Accessed 23 jul 2012

[f] Organización Mundial de la Salud (OMS) (2011). *Estadísticas sanitarias mundiales 2011.* http://www.who.int/whosis/whostat/ES_WHS2011_Full.pdf. Accessed 24 jul 2012

[g] Ministerio da Saúde, Departamento de Informática do Sistema Único de Saúde. (DATASUS). *Informações de Saúde.* http://tabnet.datasus.gov.br/cgi/tabcgi.exe?ibge/cnv/popuf.def. Accessed 18 jul 2012

[h] Departamento Nacional de Estadística (DANE). *Indicadores de mortalidad Colombia DANE, proyecciones anuales de población por sexo y edad Estudios censales 1985–2015.* Bogotá: Autor. http://www.dane.gov.co/index.php?option=com_content&view=article&id=75&Itemid=72. Accessed 18 jul 2012

[i] Así vamos en Salud (s. f.). *Indicadores de estado de salud. Tasa de mortalidad infantil.* Bogotá: Autor. http://www.asivamosensalud.org/index.php?option=com_content&view=article&id=95:tasa-de-mortalidad-infantil&catid=55:Indicadores&Itemid=74. Accessed 18 jul 2012

[j] Pan American Health Organization (PAHO). *Basic indicators country profile.* http://ais.paho.org/phip/viz/cip_maternalandinfantmortality.asp. Accessed 22 jul 2012

[k] Becerril-Montekio, V., Medina, G., & Aquino, R. (2011). The health system of Brazil. *Salud Pública Méx,* 53 (suppl 2), S120-S131

[l] Gobierno de Chile, Ministerio de Salud. (s. f.). *Defunciones y Mortalidad Materna, según región. Chile 2000–2009.* Chile: Autor. http://deis.minsal.cl/vitales/mortalidad_materna/Mortalidad_Materna2000-2009.htm. Accessed 17 jul 2012

[m] Rodríguez, H. (s. f.) *Sistema de vigilancia de Mortalidad Materna con base en la Web. Presentación realizada por OPS Colombia en el Encuentro Nacional sobre Maternidad Segural.* Ministerio de la Protección Social, el Fondo de Población de las Naciones Unidas, la Organización Panamericana de la Salud/Organización Mundial de la Salud. http://www.slideshare.net/OPSColombia/sistema-de-vigilancia-de-mortalidad-materna-con-base-en-la-web-ops-dr-hernn-rodrguez. Accessed 18 jul 2012

[n] Organización Panamericana de la Salud (OPS). (s. f.) *Indicadores básicos situación de salud* 2010. Washington: Autor. http://new.paho.org/col/index.php?option=com_content&view=article&id=25&Itemid=135. Accessed 22 jul 2012

[o] Asi vamos en Salud (s.f.). *Indicadores de estado de salud. Razón de mortalidad materna.* Bogotá: Autor. http://www.asivamosensalud.org/index.php?option=com_content&view=article&id=240:razon-mortalidad-materna&catid=55:Indicadores&Itemid=74. Accessed 18 jul 2012

[p] Presidencia de la República Mexicana, CONAPO, INEGI. Sistema de información de los objetivos de desarrollo del milenio. México: Autor. http://www.objetivosdedesarrollodelmilenio.org.mx/cgi-win/ODM.exe/ANOODM005000100010,26,DxA210144483486,000,1990,False,False,False,False,False,False,False,0,0. Accessed 26 jul 2012

Sources: See list of references al the end of the chapter

Table 3.5 Main causes of death in five Latin American countries

	1990		2007	
Country	Cause	Mortality rate per 100,000	Cause	Mortality rate per 100,000
Argentina (see table footnote f of Table 1)	SD	SD	Diseases of the circulatory system	30.2
	SD	SD	Malignant tumours	18.3
	SD	SD	Diseases of the circulatory system	15.3
	SD	SD	External causes	6.2
	SD	SD	Infectious and parasitic diseases, septicaemia	4.6
	1990		2005	
Brazil	Diseases of the circulatory system (see table footnote k of Table 4)	31.9	Diseases of the circulatory system (see table footnote b of Table 1)	28.3
	Neoplasm	15.2	Other causes	15.9
	External causes	14.6	Neoplasm	14.7
	Diseases of the respiratory system	10.9	External causes	12.5
	Infectious and parasitic diseases	5.5	Ill-defined causes	10.3
	1990		2009	
Chile[a]	Diseases of the circulatory system	26.4	Diseases of the circulatory system	27.0
	Malignant tumours	18.1	Malignant tumours	25.6
	Diseases of the respiratory system	12.3	Diseases of the respiratory system	9.7
	External causes	12.2	External causes	8.9
	Diseases of the digestive system	7.8	Diseases of digestive system	7.3
	1990		2008	
Colombia[b]	Aggression (homicide)	68.7	Ischaemic heart disease	57.1
	Ischaemic heart disease	45.3	Aggression (homicide)	41.0
	Cerebrovascular diseases	27.0	Cerebrovascular diseases	30.0
	Heart failure	17.3	Chronic disease of the respiratory system	21.6
	Pneumonia	14.8	Diabetes mellitus	15.7

(continued)

Table 3.5 (continued)

Country	1990 Cause	Mortality rate per 100,000	2007 Cause	Mortality rate per 100,000
	1995		2010	
Mexico	Diseases of the circulatory system	109.3[c]	Diabetes mellitus[d]	73.8
	External causes, injury and poisoning	63.9	Ischaemic heart disease	63.1
	Diseases of the endocrine glands	59.4	Cerebrovascular diseases	28.7
	Malignant tumours	56.2	Cirrhosis and other chronic liver diseases	25.2
	Diseases of the respiratory system	48.2	Aggression (homicide)	22.9

[a]Gobierno de Chile, Ministerio de Salud. (s. f.). *Diez primeras causas de defunción en Ambos Sexos, Chile 2000–2009*. Chile: Autor. http://www.deis.cl/estadisticas-mortalidad/. Accessed 18 jul 2012

[b]Asi vamos en Salud (s.f.). *Seguimiento al sector salud en Colombia. Indicadores de seguimientos al sector salud en Colombia. 15 diciembre 2008*. Bogotá: Autor. http://www.asivamosensalud.org/index.php. Accessed 18 jul 2012

[c]Sistema Nacional de Información en Salud. (SINAIS). (s.f.). *Efectos del cambio de la 9ª a la 10ª Revisión de la Clasificación Internacional de Enfermedades en las Estadísticas de Mortalidad en México: exploración General*. http://sinais.salud.gob.mx/descargas/pdf/SE06_EfectosCambiosCIE9a-10arev.pdf. Accessed 18 jul 2012

[d]Mexicomaxico (s. f.). *México, principales causas de mortalidad desde 1938*. www.mexico-maxico.org/Voto/MortalidadCausas.htm. Accessed 18 jul 2012

Source: See list of references al the end of the chapter

diseases became more relevant, which is also related to the increase of life expectancy, among other factors. In Colombia, assaults and homicides still occupy an important place, due to the armed conflict.

Findings of Studies Related to the Health Process

Argentina

Several studies state that the reforms undertaken since the 1990s have reproduced a segmented system focused on cost containment and have not improved access of the poor to health care (Danani s.f.; Almeida 2002). It has been argued that the public offering indirectly subsidises inefficiencies in other subsectors (Belló and Becerril 2011). To the poor articulation of the sectors, it is added unequal funding levels and quality of care and access barriers (mainly economic) for some population groups are added (Belmartino 2005:155–171). A study carried out in Cordoba, Argentina, concluded that some of the worst features of the previous health system have deepened: fragmentation, disintegration, irrationality in the use of resources, lack of coordination, funding problems and strengthening of the traditional medical model. Also new problems have emerged, such as "clientelisation" of the health sector, lack of health information, conflicts between provinces and the arbitrary closure of some services. Each municipality builds its own health responses to their problems, generating heterogeneity and fragmentation, which makes the coordination from the central level more complex. These results suggest that is not a policy to achieve greater efficiency, effectiveness, quality and participation in the health field (Ase 2006:214–216).

Brazil

Democratic participation and movements of civil society in the policy definition, management and execution control have been a key element of SUS development (CONASS 2007). It has had positive impacts as expanding service offerings increases the technical basis for public health management. Although universal coverage is one of the purposes of SUS, there is still a lot of work to do in order to achieve greater coverage and higher quality of care for all users (Silva 2009:6).

The primary health-care strategy has had great results in Brazil. One example of this approach has been a programme of nurse-directed auxiliary health workers in Ceará, a poor state in the Northeast of Brazil, which has, since 1987, served about 5 million mainly rural people. The auxiliaries, called "agentes de saúde", live in the local communities that they serve and should visit each home once a month to carry out a number of priority health activities. A key aspect of the system is timely and comprehensive information, which is based on agent visits and is managed by trained nurses (Svitone et al. 2000: 293). The Program of Family Health has been successful, with an increase from 14 to 60 % coverage of primary health services of the population and approximately 13 % reduction in infant mortality for the years 1999–2004 (Becerril et al. 2011:10; CONASS 2003; Macinko et al. 2006: 13–19). The new challenges of SUS are as follows: a) overcome the financing difficulties, b) manage dispute divergent interests between groups, c) overcome low management capacity of human resources, d) control the excessive bureaucracy, e) insufficient legal mechanisms for the regulation of private care (Silva 2009:6) and f) consolidation of decentralization in large municipalities, as a political process (Spedo et al. 2009:1).

Chile

The National Study on Satisfaction and Health Expenditure in Chile carried out in 2005 showed that the degree of user satisfaction with the health system is generally good, with an approval rating around 80 %, without significant differences among the beneficiaries from the public and private sectors (Ministerio de Salud de Chile 2007). Satisfaction levels are good in both ambulatory care and hospitalisation. Knowledge of medical and other professionals, as well as the adequacy of treatment received by the patients, is very well tested by almost all the respondents. The most critical aspects were, firstly, the waiting time for outpatient care once the person reached the settlement, which was considered too long or longer by 29 % of users, and, secondly, the treatment of staff (Becerril et al. 2011:141).

The municipal health experience is very different in the financial, human and leadership skills; therefore, it does not seem appropriate to implement a generalised model of decentralization in all municipalities. Sometimes, some municipalities have achieved cooperation partners in the health sector, with some significant successes. Coordination with hospitals and the provision of quality professional resources constitute important difficulties to municipal primary health (Galilea et al. 2011). A study carried out in Colombia and Chile suggests that decentralization, under certain conditions and with some specific policy mechanisms, can contribute to, or at least maintain, more equitable allocation of health resources among municipalities. The data from Colombia show that a population-based formula for national allocations is an effective mechanism for achieving equity of expenditures. Evidence from these countries also suggests that more equitable allocation of resources may contribute to more equitable utilisation of health services across income groups (Bossert et al. 2003:99).

Colombia

Several studies have found limitation in the administrative capacity of the Colombian municipalities to manage health sector in spite of the certification, which was awarded because of political pressure rather than for having technical capacity (Molina et al. 2011; Granados and Gómez 2000; Ministerio de Salud de Colombia 2001); there are no clear-cut differences between certified and non-certified municipalities in relation to their administrative capacity (Pinto et al. 2005:149; Molina 2009a). Other studies have showed limited development or lack of a planning process and weak health information system (Departamento Nacional de Planeación 1999:5–6; Granados and Gómez 2000:9, Molina 2009a; Molina et al. 2011) and low qualification of the staff at all governmental levels, which have suffered from a high turnover because of the political patronage that has undermined its institutional capacity and leadership (World Bank 1998:5; Bossert et al. 1998; Molina 2009b; Molina et al. 2011). Homedes and Ugalde (2011:498) argue that with decentralization, decisions based on political criteria continue to hinder the implementation of improvements with allocative efficiency. Likewise, the lack of a precise relationship between funding and the population served creates perverse incentives that often add grantees—people politically close to those in power (Galilea 2011: 142).

In public health issues, there has been a deterioration of the disease prevention programmes and epidemiological surveillance due to the disintegration of the network of institutions (Granados and Gómez 2000; Molina et al. 2011; Estevens 2012). There has been a re-emergence of transmissible diseases previously controlled (Yadon et al. 2006: 21–23). With the implementation of the Social Security System, the key health indicators and disease control programmes have deteriorated. The explanation lies in the inefficiency of contracting out; the weak economic, technical and political capacity of the Colombian government to regulate and control; and the absence of real participation of the poor in health policy decision-making (De Groote et al. 2005). In addition, several studies have showed weak development of community participation (Ministerio de Salud de Colombia 2001; Herrera 1999:9; Mosquera et al. 2001; Molina 2009a:15) due to (a) lack of specific resources; (b) participation is tied to predetermined procedures; (c) private sector discouragement with the organisation of user's associations; and (d) community leaders had limited knowledge on health issues and their entitlements.

With the simultaneous implementation of health decentralization and the SSSH, which encouraged privatisation and market economy, people have to tackle several new administrative, economic and geographical barriers and problems with accessibility and quality of the health services (Vargas and Molina 2009; Molina 2009a).

Mexico

A study carried out in Baja California (México, 1996–2004) showed that decentralization of the health sector has not improved the supply of services; the waiting time to get a medical consultation increased; the population without health insurance has not received benefits of decentralization, related to better accessibility, equity and quality of services (Jaramillo 2007b:503–504). Also, the municipalities did not overcome the dependency of the central government (Jaramillo 2007a:85). Another study carried out by Homedes and Ugalde (2011) in six Mexican states (Baja California Sur, Colima, Guanajuato, Nuevo León, Sonora y Tamaulipas) concluded that the decentralization's objectives were not achieved. Only in Guanajuato and Nuevo Leon did efficiency improved through inter-institutional coordination mechanisms. Equity has not improved because the poorest regions hardly capture human and financial resources. The imposition of fees for services has created financial barriers in accessibility to services in the poorest populations. Homedes and Ugalde (2011:498–499) found that central government continues to award funds based on historical budgets, and therefore, the more developed states receive more. The process is at fault due to the following: (a) responded to pressures and specific interests of the World Bank and the International Monetary Fund, which do not coincide with national and local interests; (b) lack of staff training at the sub-national levels; (c) unclear functions of each administrative level; (d) lack of policies for equitable distribution of resources and protection of vulnerable populations; and (e) lack of consensus with the different political groups, especially the opposition to ensure policy continuity (Homedes and Ugalde (2011:501–502). The Mexican health reforms have not resulted in significant reductions of health inequities, or in increased efficiency, productivity or quality, despite their costs (Homedes and Ugalde 2009).

Finally, a literature review carried out by Ugalde and Homedes (2008:47–49) about health in LACs concluded that community participation has not increased; there is no evidence of the relationship between decentralization and better democracy. Efficiency has not improved because of the lack of quality of staff, related to patronage system, more local and central bureaucracy and lack of economy of scale strategies, among others. There is no evidence of improving quality of services with decentralization.

Discussion

Decentralization has been implemented using different approaches in each country, and therefore, there should be different results and impacts related to efficiency, equity and quality in the provision of services, financial resources distribution, community participation and public health indicators (Jaramillo 2007b:496). But in the LACs analysed, decentralization of the health sector was introduced simultaneously with privatisation, within a context of a neoliberal economic model, emphasising financial issues (Ase 2006:214). In some countries, privatisation, separation and fragmentation of stewardship, insurance and provision functions and institutions; intermediation; and competitive market between health institutions have made the health systems very complex, affecting the provision of services, especially public health programmes that do not represent financial profitability to the private sector. The private sector looks for its own interest rather than for the accomplishment of the public functions transferred by the governments. So the market failures of privatisation affect the results of decentralization. These aspects make the health process very complex and difficult to analyse as also appointed Bankauskaite and Saltman (2007:11–21). Galilea et al. (2011) argue that domination of privatisation and the selective and targeted policies put in place simultaneously could explain the difficulties to implement universal coverage and the strengthening of health systems at the provincial and municipal levels. Brazil could be an exception to this, because the SUS is funded by general taxes, not in contributory scheme to private and public insurers, and the MOH and the municipal and states authorities lead the system; so Brazil seems to have a better structure of its decentralised health system. Rather than in the Colombian experience, the private insurers interfere and overlap the functions of the Ministry of Health, affecting stewardship of the health system and its process. What would happen if the decentralization of health were implemented without mixing it with privatisation? Perhaps the results would be better.

In the Colombian case, during the operation of the National Health System (1974–1990), several national health plans were put in place, and there was a positive impact on the control and prevention of diseases, a decrease in infant mortality rate (from 44 per 1,000 live births in 1975–1980 to 21 per 1,000 live births in 1995–2000) and maternal mortality rates and the main public health indicators (Departamento Nacional de Planeación 2002).

With decentralization and the Social Security System involving privatisations, competitive market among insurers, providers, etc., the preventive public health programmes were discouraged in the hospitals and some were closed and the expert public health staff was reduced or replaced by non-qualified staff in order to decrease costs (Málaga et al. 2000; Martinez et al. 2001, Molina et al. 2011), and consequently public health indicators reversed (Esteves 2012:2). This situation is contrary to the importance of the capacity and availability of human resources at all governmental levels to the decentralization process, especially at the municipal level (Mills 1990; Yadón et al. 2006: 20). Jaramillo (1997) argues that the focus of Law 100 of 1993 was not public health; instead, it has emphasised individuals and curative health services.

With health decentralization, political parties have been more involved within the health institutions and decision-making, which has affected negatively the technical capacity of the public health sector due to its influence in allocating resources based on the interests of the rolling group, rather than on community needs, and also because of the influence in quality and stability of human resources, linked to patronage system. In this sense, Bossert (2000:1) suggested that with decentralization, local decision-making is influenced by patronage and nepotism that affect the performance of human resources. How can we prevent interference of political parties within health institutions to improve their institutional capability and performance? How could we harmonise decentralization policies with labour reforms to improve the institutional capacity of the health sector? What are the practical possibilities that decentralization improves coverage, accessibility and quality of health services? What have been the effects of decentralization and privatisation on public health policies and programmes?

The studies carried out on health in these five countries have had very different objectives and analytical framework; therefore, it is difficult to compare them. There is a need to develop a unified analytical approach to study decentralization, in order to carry out comparative international analysis. Also, the governments and the academic sector should carry out national debates on decentralization and evaluate its achievements, limitations and perspectives.

Recommended Readings

Yadón, S., Gürtler, R., Tobar F. & Medici, A. (2006) *Descentralización y control de enfermedades trasmisibles en América Latina*. Organización Panamericana de la Salud; Banco Interamericano de Desarrollo, Universidad de Buenos Aires. Buenos Aires.

This book is focused on decentralization and public health programmes and presents an evaluation of the decentralization on the transmissible disease programmes in Latin American countries. This also highlights the situation of the management of transmissible disease programme and compares their vertical and horizontal approaches.

Saltman, R., Bankauskaite, V., & Vrangbaek, K. (2007). *Decentralization in health Care. European observatory on health system and policies series*. New York: World Health Organization.

This book explores the capacity and impact of decentralization within the European health-care systems. It examines both the theoretical underpinnings and recent practical experiences, drawing upon both published literature and evidence collected directly from the field. The book also assesses the appropriateness of management processes within the health system for implementing a successful decentralization strategy.

Acknowledgements We are very grateful with Dr Krishna Regmi because he invited us to write this chapter for this book.

References

ABRASCO, CEBES, ABRES, REDE UNIDA, AMPASA. O SUS para valer: *universal, humanizado e de qualidade*. http://www.cebes.org.br/media/file/O%20SUS%20PRA%20VALER%20REDUZIDO%20(10jul2006).pdf. Accessed on 21 oct 2010.

Aquino, R., Oliveira, N. F., & Barreto, M. L. (2009). Impact of the Family Health Program on infant mortality in Brazilian municipalities. *American Journal of Public Health, 99*(1), 87–93.

Ase, I. (2006). La Descentralizaci6n de Servicios de Salud en Córdoba (Argentina): Entre la Confianza Democrática y el Desencanto Neoliberal. *Salud colectiva, 2*(2), 199–218.

Bahia, L. (2005). Padrões e mudanças no financiamento e regulação do Sistema de Saúde Brasileiro: impactos sobre as relações entre o público e privado. *Saude Soc, 14*(2), 9–30.

Bankauskaite, V., & Saltman, R. (2007), Central issues in decentralization debate. In Saltman, R., Bankauskaite, V., & Vrangbaek, K. (2007). *Decentralization in health Care. European Observatory on Health System and Policies Series*. New York: World Health Organization

Barros, E. (2003). *Financiamento do Sistema de Saúde no Brasil: marco legal e comportamento do gasto*. Brasflia: Organização Pan-Americana da Saúde.

Barros, M. A. D., & Porto, S. M. (2008). Financiamento e alocação de recursos em saúde no Brasil. In: Giovanella, L. (Org.). *Políticas e sistemas de saúde no Brasil*. Rio de Janeiro: FIOCRUZ

Batley, R. (1996). Public–private relationships and performance in service provision. *Urban Studies, 33*(4–5), 723–751.

Becerril, V., Medina, G., & Aquino, R. (2011a). Sistema de salud de Brasil. *Salud Pública de México, 53*(Suppl 2), 120–131.

Becerril, V., Reyes, J. D., & Manuel, A. (2011b). Sistema de salud de Chile. *Salud Pública de México, 53*(Suppl 2), 132–153.

Bell6, M., & Becerril, V. (2011). Sistema de salud de Argentina. *Salud Pública de México, 53*(Suppl 2), 5.

Belmartino, S. (2005). Una década de reforma de la atenci6n médica en Argentina. *Salud Colectiva, 21*, 155–171.

Bermudez, J. A. Z., Oliveira, M. A., & Luiza, V. L. (2008). Asistencia farmacêutica. In L. Giovanella, S. Escorel, L. V. C. Lobato, J. C. Noronha, & A. I. Carvalho (Eds.), *Políticas e sistemas de saúde no Brasil* (pp. 435–472). Rio de Janeiro: FIOCRUZ.

Bossert, T., Hsiao, W., Barrera, M., Alarcon, L., Leo, M., & Caseres, C. (1998). Transformation of ministries of health in the area of health reform: The case of Colombia. *Health Policy and Planning, 13*(1), 59–77.

Bossert, T., Larrañaga, O., Giedion, U., Arbelaez, J., & Bowser, M. (2003). Decentralization and equity of resource allocation: Evidence from Colombia and Chile. *Bulletin of the World Health Organization, 81*(2), 95–100.

Bossert, T. (2000). La Descentralizaci6n de los Sistemas de Salud en Latinoamérica: u análisis comparativo de Chile. Colombia y Bolivia. *Health Sector Reform Iniciative, 29.*

Burki, S. J. (1999). Globalization to Localization. In S. J. Burki, G. Perry, F. Eid, M. Freire, V. Vergara, & S. Webb (Eds.), *Annual World Bank Conference on Development in Latin America and the Caribbean, 1999: Decentralization and Accountability of the Public Sector* (pp. 3–5). Washington: The World Bank.

Castañeda, T., Beeharry, G., & Griffin, C. (1999). Decentralization of health services in Latin American Countries: Issues and some lessons. In S. J. Burki, G. Perry, F. Eid, M. Freire, V. Vergara, & S. Webb (Eds.), *Annual World Bank Conference on Development in Latin America and the Caribbean, 1999: Decentralization and accountability of the public sector* (pp. 249–272). Washington: The World Bank.

Collins, C. D., Omar, M & Tarín E. (2002). Decentralization, health care and policy process in the Punjab, Pakistan in the 1990s. Recuperado el 18 de julio de 2012 en www.intercience.wiley.com.

Collins, C. D., Araujo, J., & Barbosa, J. (2000). Decentralizing the health sector: issues in Brazil. *Health Policy, 52*, 113–127.

Conselho Nacional de Secretários de Saúde (CONASS). (2003). *A saúde na opinião dos brasileiros. Um estudio prospectivo.* Brasilia: Autor. http://www.conass.org.br/admin/arquivos/opiniao_brasileiros1.pdf. Accessed 18 may 2010.

Conselho Nacional de Secretários de Saúde (CONASS). (2007). *Regulação em Saúde. Brasília: CONASS.* http://dtr2004saude.gov.br/dab/docs/publicacoes/conass_progestores/livro_10_ regulacao_em_saude.pdf. Accessed 12 aug 2010.

Collins, C., & Green, A. (1993). Decentralization and primary health care in developing countries: Ten key questions. *Journal of Management in Medicine, 7*(2), 58–68.

Danani, C. (s. f). *Los procesos que esconde la reforma de la seguridad social en Argentina. El caso de las Obras Sociales.* Buenos Aires: Instituto de Investigaciones Gino Germani, Facultad de Ciencias Sociales, Universidad de Buenos Aires.

De Groote, T., De Paepe, P., & Unger, J. P. (2005). Colombia: In vivo test of health sector privatization in the developing world. *International Journal of Health Services, 35*(1), 124–141.

Departamento Nacional de Planeación (DNP). (1999). *Informe de Desarrollo Humano para Colombia.* Bogotá: Tercer Mundo Editores.

Departamento Nacional de Planeación (DNP). (2002). *Evaluación del a descentralización en Colombia.* Bogotá: Autor.

Enthoven, A.C. (1985). National Health Service: some reforms that might be politically feasible. In: Mullen, P. (1998) Planning and Internal Market. In: Spurgeon, P. (Eds.) (1998) *The New Face of the NHS.* London: The Royal Society of Medicine Press Ltd.

Esteves, R. (2012). The quest for equity in Latin America: A comparative analysis of the health care reforms in Brazil and Colombia. *International Journal for Equity in Health, 11*, 6.

Exworthy, M., & Halford, S. (2002). *Professionals and the New Managerialism in the Public Sector.* Buckingham: Open University Press.

Franco, S. (1993). Teoría y práctica de la Salud Pública. *Revista Facultad Nacional Salud PÚBLICA, 12*(2), 63–76.

Fundación Mexicana para la Salud (FUNSALUD). (2012). *La Salud en México, 2006–2012.* México, D. F.: Visión de FUNSALUD

Galilea, S., Letelier, L., & Ross, K. (2011). *Descentralización de servicios esenciales. Los casos de Brasil, Chile, Colombia, Costa Rica y México en salud, educación, residuos, seguridad y fomento.* Nueva York: Comisión Económica para América Latina y el Caribe (CEPAL), Naciones Unidas.

Gómez-Dantés, O., Sesma, S., Becerril, V. M., Knaul, F. M., Arreola, H., & Frenk, J. (2011). Sistema de salud de México. *Salud Pública de México, 53*(S2), 220–232.

Granados, R. T., & Gómez, M. C. (2000). La reforma de los sistemas de salud en Chile y Colombia: Resultados y balance. *Rev Salud Pública, 2*(2), 97–120.

Griffiths, R. and Crump, C. (1998). A public Health Perspective. In Spurgeon P. (ed) (1998). The Face of the NHS. The Royal Sociaty of Medicine Press Ltd., London.

Guimarães, J. A. (2004). A pesquisa médica e biomédica no Brasil. Comparações com o desempenho científico brasileiro e mundial. *Ciência e Saúde Coletiva, 9*(2), 303–327.

Herrera, V. (1999). Régimen Subsidiado de Salud: Evolución y Problemática. *Rev Salud Pública, 1*(3), 193–211.

Homedes, N., & Ugalde ,A., (Eds.). (2006). *Decentralizing health services in México. A case study in state reform*. California: The University of California, Center for U.S.-Mexican Studies.

Homedes, N., & Ugalde, A. (2009). Twenty-five years of convoluted health reforms in Mexico. *PLoS Medicine, 6*(8), e1000124.

Homedes, N., & Ugalde, A. (2011). Descentralización de los servicios de salud: estudios de caso en seis estados mexicanos. *Salud Pública de México, 53*(6), 493–503.

Islam, A., & Tahir, M. Z. (2002). Health sector reform in South Asia: New Challenges and constrains. *Health Policy, 60*, 151–169.

Jaramillo, M. C. (2007a). La descentralización de la salud en México. Avances y retrocesos. *Rev. Gerencia Políticas Salud, 6*(13), 85–111.

Jaramillo, M. C. (2007b). La descentralización del sector salud en México: el caso de Baja California. *Rev Salud Pública, 9*(4), 495–505.

Jaramillo, I. (1997). *Descentralización del Sector Salud. Una década de descentralización en*. Bogotá: Colombia.

Kutzin, J. (1995). *Experience with organizational and financing reform of the health Sector*. Geneva: World Health Organization.

Legemaate, J. (2002). Integrating health law and health policy: A European perspective. *Health Policy, 60*, 101–110.

Londoño, B., Jaramillo, I., & Uribe, J. P. (1999). *Descentralización y Reforma en los Servicios de Salud: El Caso Colombiano*. Bogotá: Banco Mundial.

López, M. R. (1995). *Fiscal Decentralization in Latin America*. Washington, D.C.: The World Bank.

Macinko, J., Guanais, F., & Marinho, M. (2006). Evaluation of the impact of the Family Health Program on infant mortality in Brazil, 1990–2002. *Journal of Epidemiology and Community Health, 60*, 13–19.

Málaga, H., Latorre, M. C., Cárdenas, J., Montiel, H., Sampson, C., Taborda, M. C., Granados, R., & Pastor, D. (2000). Equidad y Reforma en Salud en Colombia. *Rev Salud Pública, 2*(3), 193–219.

Martínez, P., Rodríguez, L. A., & Agudelo, C. (2001). Equidad en la Política de Reforma del Sistema de Salud. *Rev Salud Pública, 3*(1), 13–39.

Mascareño, C. (1996). *Municipalización de los Servicios Sociales en América Latina*. Caracas: CLAD.

Mills, A., Bennett, S., & Russel, S. (2001). *The challenge of health sector reform. What must government do?* New York: Palgrave.

Mills, A., Vaughan, J., Smith, D., & Tabibzadeh, I. (1990). *Health system decentralization. Concepts, issues and country experience*. Geneva: World Health Organization.

Ministério da Saúde. (2006). *Diretrizes para a implantação de complexos reguladores*. Brasília: Ministério da Saúde. Secretaria de Atenção à Saúde, Departamento de Regulação, Avaliação e Controle de Sistemas. http://portal.saude.gov.br/portal/arquivos/pdf/pactovolume6.pdf. Accessed 2 oct 2010.

Ministerio de Salud de Chile. (2007). *Estudio Nacional sobre Satisfacción y Gasto en Salud. Informe de Resultados*: *satisfacción con el sistema de salud*. Chile: Autor. http://epi.minsal.cl/epi/html/invest/ENSG/Informe_final_Satisfaccion.pdf. Accessed 2 jun 2010.

Ministerio de Salud de Colombia. (2001). *Municipio Centinela: Evaluación del a implementación del Sistema General de Seguridad en Salud. 1997 – 1999*. Bogotá: Autor.

Molina, G., Ramírez, A., & Muñoz, I. (Eds.). (2011). *Dilemas en las decisiones en la atención en salud. Ética, derechos y deberes constitucionales frente a la rentabilidad financiera en el sistema de salud colombiano* (2nd ed.). Bogotá: Editorial La Carreta.

Molina, G. (2009a). An integrity perspective on the decentralization of the health sector in Colombia. *Forum Qualitative Social Research, 10*(2), 1–28.

Molina, G. (2009b). Rol de los partidos políticos en la provisión de servicios de salud, Colombia 2007–2008. *Revista Facultad Nacional De Salud Pública, 27*(1), 66–75.

Molina, G., Rodríguez, C., Montoya, N., & Spurgeon, P. (2006). Descentralización del sector salud en Colombia, Análisis de 91 municipios. *Revista Facultad Nacional de Salud Pública, 24*(1), 48–60.

Mosquera, M., Zapata, Y., Lee, K., Arango, C., & Varela, A. (2001). Strengthen user participation through health sector reform in Colombia: a study of institutional change and social representation. *Health Policy and Planning, 16*(Suppl 2), 52–60.

MSAS. (1994). *Boletín epidemiológico nacional No. 2*. Buenos Aires: Autor.

Nigenda, G., & Machado, M. H. (2000). From State to market: The Nicaraguan labour market for health personnel. *Health Policy and Planning, 15*(3), 312–318.

Organización Panamericana de la Salud. (2001). *Perfiles de los Sistemas de Salud. Perfil de los sistemas y servicios de salud de Argentina* (2nd ed.). Washington, DC: Autor.

Organización Panamericana de la Salud. (2005). *Perfil del sistema de salud de Brasil*. Brasilia: Autor.

Organización Panamericana de la Salud (OPS). (2007). *La Renovación de la Atención Primaria de Salud en las Américas*. Washington DC: Autor.

Organización Mundial de la Salud (OMS). (2008). *Informe final de la Comisión OMS sobre los determinantes sociales de la salud*. Ginebra: Autor.

Pinto, D., Carrasquilla, G., Gil, F., Collazos, C., & Rincón, J. (2005). La certificación como un indicador de descentralización en salud. Una mirada a la luz del cumplimiento de requisitos en municipios colombianos. *Rev. Gerencia y Política de Salud, 8*, 149–162.

Pollitt, C., Birchall, J., & Putman, K. (1998). *Decentralizing Public Service Management*. London: Macmillan Press Ltd.

Rivas, P. (s. f). La descentralización de la provisión de servicios de salud. Washington D.C.: OPS. http://www.paho.org/spanish/dpm/shd/hp/hp-x-taller03-rivas.pdf. Accessed 11 nov 2010.

Reyes, J., & Annick, M. (2011). Sistema de salud de Chile. *Salud Pública de México, 53*(Suppl 2), 132–153.

Rojas, F. (1999). The political context of decentralization in Latin America. In S. J. Burki, G. Perry, F. Eid, M. Freire, V. Vergara, & S. Webb (Eds.), *Annual World Bank Conference on Development in Latin America and the Caribbean, 1999: Decentralization and accountability of the public sector* (pp. 9–32). Washington: The World Bank.

Rondinelli, D. A. (1990). *Decentralizing Urban Development Programs: A framework for analyzing Policy options*. Washington, D.C.: US. Agency for International Development, Office of Housing.

Rothstein, M. (2002). Rethinking the meaning of public health. *The Journal of Law, Medicine & Ethics, 30*(2), 144–149.

Sarmiento, A. (2004). *La institucionalidad social en Colombia: la búsqueda de una descentralización como centro*. Santiago de Chile: CEPAL. División de Desarrollo Social.

Scott, C. (2001). *Public and private roles in health care systems*. Buckingham: Open University Press.

Silva, M. T. (2009). Sistema Único de Salud: La Experiencia Brasileña en la Universalización del acceso a la Salud. *Revista Peruana de Medicina Experimental y Salud Pública, 26*(2), 251–257.

Smith, P. C., Stepan, A., Valdmanis, V., & Verheyen, P. (1997). Principal-agent problems in health care systems: An international perspective. *Health Policy, 41*(1), 37–60.

Spedo, S. M., Tanaka, O. Y., & Rodrigues da Silva, N. O. (2009). Desafio da descentralização do Sistema Único de Saúde em município de grande porte: o caso de São Paulo. *Brasil Cad Saúde Pública, 25*(8), 1781–1790.

Superintendencia de Servicios de Salud (2010). *Carta Compromiso*. Buenos Aires. Argentina: Autor. http://www.sssalud.gov.ar/institucion/archivos/carta_com.pdf. Accessed 1 jul 2010.

Svitone, E. C., Garfield, R., Vasconcelos, M. I., & Craveiro, V. A. (2000). Primary health care lessons from the Northeast of Brazil: The Agentes de Saúde Program. *Revista Panamericana de Salud Pública, 7*(5), 293–302.

Teixeira, M. G., & Costa, M. C. N. (2008). Vigilância epidemiológica: políticas, sistemas e serviços. En: Giovanella, L. (Org.). *Políticas e sistemas de saúde no Brasil*. Rio de Janeiro: FIOCRUZ.

The World Bank. (1997). *World Development Report 1997. The State in a Changing World.* New York: The International Bank for Reconstruction and Development/The World Bank, Oxford University Press.
The World Bank. (2001). *World Development Report 2000/2001: Attacking Poverty*. New York: Oxford University Press.
The World Bank/Banco Interamericano de Desarrollo. (1998). *Decentralización en Colombia.* Nuevos Desafíos. RE3-98-002. Washington D.C.: The World Bank.
Thomason, J. A., Newbrander, W. C., & Riitta-Liisa, K. (1991). *Decentralization in developing countries: The experience of Papua New Guinea and its health service*. Geneva: WHO, National Centre for Development Studies.
Ugalde, A., & Homedes, N. (2008). La descentralización de los servicios de salud: de la teoría a la práctica. *Rev Salud Colectiva, 4*(1), 31–56.
Vargas, J., & Molina, G. (2009). Acceso a los servicios de salud en seis ciudades de Colombia: limitaciones y consecuencias. *Revista Facultad Nacional De Salud Pública, 27*(2), 121–130.
Vergara, M., & Martínez, M. S. (2006). Financiamiento del sistema de salud chileno. *Salud Pública de México, 48*(6), 512–521.
World Health Organization (WHO). (1998). *Athens declaration for healthy cities*. Athens: Autor.
Yadón, S., Gürtler, R., Tobar, F., & Medici, A. (2006). *Descentralización y control de enfermedades trasmisibles en América Latina*. Buenos Aires: Organización Panamericana de la Salud, Banco Interamericano de Desarrollo, Universidad de Buenos Aires.

Chapter 4
Decentralization and Governance in Health Care

Norman Flynn

Abstract This chapter examines the relationship between decentralization and governance processes. It first reviews the fiscal federalism argument that decentralization will produce positive results both in productive efficiency and in allocative efficiency by establishing more direct accountability and by promoting competition. It then turns to a conventional and narrow definition of governance, the choice of mechanisms through which actions and behaviours of individuals and organisations are governed, and asks how decentralization can be carried out within each governance mechanism. The wider term 'good governance' and the impact of decentralization on it is treated next, with the argument that both centralised and decentralised systems can exhibit characteristics of good and bad governance. Three case studies, Spain, Poland and Indonesia, are used to illustrate different aspects of decentralization and governance.

After Reading This Chapter You Will Be Able To

- *Understand the main reasons put forward for decentralization*
- *Define productive and allocative efficiency*
- *Know the impact of decentralization in a range of governance mechanisms*
- *Explain the impact of decentralization in three different case examples*

N. Flynn (✉)
SOAS, University of London, London, UK
e-mail: nf17@soas.ac.uk

K. Regmi (ed.), *Decentralizing Health Services: A Global Perspective*,
DOI 10.1007/978-1-4614-9071-5_4, © Springer Science+Business Media New York 2014

Introduction: Fiscal Federalism

Musgrave's (1959) argument for fiscal decentralization was the intellectual foundation of a long period of decentralization in the governance of public services generally and in health care specifically. Decentralization was in fashion in Europe, the Americas, those developing countries in receipt of Official Development Assistance and with governments pursuing 'new public management' agendas until at least the decades 1980s and 1990s.

The fiscal federalism argument was that devolved financial, managerial and political controls would improve performance of public service organisations in both cost terms (productive efficiency) and in producing services that match the people's needs and preferences (allocative efficiency). In addition, competition among localities would arise as people chose where to live according to the levels and types of services available and the taxes raised to provide them.

Improvements in productive efficiency would be achieved by managers enabled to change the production function to take account of local factor costs, while improvements in allocative efficiency would arise from contact with service users enabled to express their needs and preferences which could then be responded to. Centralisation, with decisions made by remote bureaucrats and politicians out of touch with local conditions, could never achieve the same levels of efficiency and responsiveness available to local managers and elected politicians.

In addition, the exposure of managers and politicians at local level would create better accountability than that achieved by remotely located leaders. Local exposure should increase accountability and therefore responsiveness. Some commentators (e.g., Saltman et al. 2007) have detected a tendency to recentralise, especially in Europe, in more recent times. We next look at the drivers for centralisation and the tension between them and the drivers for decentralization.

Efficiency Versus Quality

There is an economic argument for centralisation: vertical integration and unified supply chains reduce transaction costs, increase government's purchasing power and thereby improve productive efficiency. Central procurement both of assets such as hospitals and consumables such as drugs would reduce overall costs compared with a devolved system with many more transactions and a more dispersed purchaser or set of purchasers. Strong vertical integration implies governance arrangements with small discretion and autonomy at lower levels of the organisation. Managers at service delivery level would use the assets and consumables, and in most cases also the staff, handed down to them, usually accompanied by a manual about how to do the job.

Counter to this argument is the idea that quality of care depends on horizontal integration, rather than vertical integration, and that where there is a multitude of service providers, effective horizontal integration can only be achieved at an organisational level close to the service user. The creation of care packages to meet individual needs and preferences can never be successfully done through the creation of a set of rules at a central level. Horizontal integration or at least co-ordination among people delivering different services implies discretion at that level about whom to work with and how.

The tension between vertical and horizontal integration and between cost efficiency and quality in business generally leads to oscillation between the two: periods of cost competition generate vertical integration along the value chain and competition based on relative quality leads to periods of searching for innovations and therefore collaborative relationships with companies with new ideas. The latter phase often results in a consolidation period of mergers and acquisitions through which the innovative companies are absorbed by the industry leaders or the innovators become the industry leaders.

This oscillation may be one explanation for the waves of decentralization and re-centralisation in health care: periods of relative fiscal looseness and therefore lower concern with the issue of cost allow experimentation in forms of care, which in turn encourage local freedom to innovate, and periods of fiscal tightening encourage an emphasis on reducing cost and therefore strengthening of central control over budgets. In any case new treatments and approaches are best developed through experimentation, which implies a high degree of discretion at local level.

Decentralising What?

The standard classification (Rondinelli 1983) of decentralization into devolution, delegation and deconcentration tries to deconstruct what we mean by decentralization. At the top level is health policy: the big decisions about the level of funding and its distribution among the various components of a health system, public health, primary care, secondary care and so on. Less strategic is the collection of revenues, through taxes and user fees to finance the health system. At the lowest level is the question of who manages the processes involved in delivering health care. Each of these three components can, in principle, be either centralised or decentralised:

	Decentralised	Centralised
Policy	Local policies, no national plan	National priorities, service design, standards
Funding	Local taxes and service charges	National taxes
Management	Local recruitment, pay scales, management arrangements. Assets acquired through local means	Nationally paid staff, central pay scales, rules and procedures, national inspection and monitoring Central asset management

The question of equity has a big influence on the choice: where both incomes and wealth and the incidence of disease are unevenly distributed, some political systems are designed to reduce the inequalities. This leads to national health policies and health funding rather than allowing big local differences. National funding and policy often imply national management and control. This applies to the equalisation of health spending per head of population, either through national taxation or through equalisation funds to bring spending in poor areas up to average levels. In many cases, it also implies a set of national minimum standards about what is to be provided and to what standard.

The acquisition and maintenance of assets are an important aspect of the choice: large, specialist hospitals are likely to serve a larger catchment area than smaller facilities and likely to be beyond the financial scope of a highly decentralised local government. Regional, provincial or national governments (depending on the scale of the country and its health system) are therefore more likely to be able to finance large-scale assets. This often leads to a mixed system of centralisation and decentralization: primary care and public health at the lost local level, with a hierarchy above the local level of regional and national facilities.

The third influence on the actual degree of decentralization of control is the nature of the employment of the medical staff. At one end of a spectrum, there are systems in which medical personnel are employees of the national government and trained in state medical schools and health facilities. Staff are allocated, with varying degrees of choice for the individuals, to posts in clinics and hospitals and remain under the managerial control of the Ministry of Health or similar body. Central management of the staff includes their remuneration, on national pay scales, their further training and development, their promotion to higher grades and their subsequent postings within the health service.

At the other end of a spectrum, there is a labour market in which individual facilities, clinics and hospitals, employ their own staff according to local agreements on pay and conditions. Employers in remote or unpopular locations may have to pay a premium salary to attract staff. There is likely to be a surplus of staff and staff of higher quality in popular locations, especially capital cities. This situation normally leads to an uneven geographical distribution of staff, of service quality and of health outcomes.

Once a policy of decentralization is adopted, clearly the real devolution of authority in a system where all medical staff are employed on central contracts will necessarily be more limited than the decentralization in free labour market systems. The case studies of Spain and Indonesia illustrate the impact of decentralization on the distribution of health-care facilities.

Decentralization and Governance

We have seen that the impact of decentralization on the Musgravian elements of productive and allocative efficiency clearly depends to some extent on what is being decentralised. It also depends on the governance arrangements that are established. Williamson's classic (1975) definition of governance mechanisms has a choice of three: the market, the hierarchy and the clan. We can add a fourth in the case of health care, governance through a network, centred on the service user. The elements of a governance structure working through a hierarchy are hierarchical supervision arrangements organised in a monocratic way, rules and procedures and employment contracts between the organisation and its employees.

The clan elements consist of professionals managing themselves, based on a shared set of values and professional skills. They do not require rules within the organisation, because their profession imbues them with a set of beliefs and behaviours through which their conduct is managed.

The market is based on a set of market transactions, in which goods and services are defined and exchanged for cash. The market consists of individual suppliers competing with each other on the basis of price and quality. A network, centred in a service user, consists of individual elements of service which the user assembles and may access through direct payments or through the exercise of entitlements to services. The entitlements may be exercised through the use of vouchers, or some administrative arrangements, sometimes mediated by a professional. Decentralization can be enacted through each of these governance mechanisms, although some are more conducive than others.

Decentralization Through Hierarchy

Decentralization within a hierarchy implies managing through rules and procedures, but pushing some of the decision-making and control to lower levels of the organisation. 'Deconcentration', or the transfer of staff from central to sub-national tiers of government, is one way of apparently decentralising administration without transferring any authority from the centre, especially when the staff transferred remain controlled by and accountable to the hierarchy and not any institutions in the locality. In the case of deconcentration, the daily management may be transferred to local level, as in France's distribution of local offices of the Ministry of Health, but decision-making on strategic maters is still centralised.

Decentralization through a hierarchy will inevitably create tensions between centre and locality over the direction of policy. Cassels (1995) reported on early efforts to decentralise while maintaining a hierarchy, with the Ministry of Finance at the top of the tree in Ghana: '…district and regional health management teams have little incentive to make efficiency savings by reducing staff numbers. If they reduce staff numbers, any savings revert to the treasury and cannot be used for non-salary costs' (p.341).

In addition to maintaining a financial hierarchy, there are various ways for central ministries to maintain professional and managerial hierarchies after an ostensible decentralization. These include prescriptive rules and procedures, inspection and audit procedures and demanding processes of planning and performance management that restrict the freedom of action of local management.

Cassels further reported on experiments with supposedly autonomous hospital boards in east Africa that 'In practice, managers have limited control over hospital resources, often remaining bound by civil service regulations despite the intention of the legislative frameworks that established the boards' (p.342). Bossert and Beauvais (2002) reported similar results in Uganda, where salaries and other major expenditures were a constraint on local discretion in budget allocation.

One way of interpreting these results is that the decentralization created increased accountability at local levels, both upwards to the hierarchy and downwards to the citizens and service users, without a concomitant increase in authority. We know that generally such an imbalance between accountability and authority cannot lead to an improvement in performance.

The other constraint on effective decentralization within a hierarchy is the capacity for decision-making and effective management at local level. Mitchell and Bossert (2010) found that both fiscal and nonfinancial resources, especially skilled and confident staff, are a constraint on the exercise of local discretion: '... some health-sector functions...require technical capacities that can far exceed what is possible at the local level, even for health-sector administrators' (p. 681).

Decentralising a Clan

The clan governance mechanism implies that individuals will behave in similar ways, wherever power and control is located: in theory a clinic or a hospital will still be run in a similar way wherever it sits in the organisation because the behaviours are determined by beliefs and training, rather than rules and incentives. It could be argued that organisational form above the level of the individual service delivery unit is irrelevant to the medical staff working there: they will continue to manage their relationship to their patients in the same way whatever management structures are in place. Tensions arise when the management structure tries to replace a clan arrangement with a hierarchy or with a market. Many medical professionals resist having their behaviour controlled or influenced by rules not of their making or by commercial imperatives of profitability.

An example of a decentralization to district level in India shows that the medical professionals were able to exert their influence at local level, despite the design of the policy at state level:

> 'The health aspects of unsafe water, wastes of the chemical industry, pesticides used in agriculture, air pollution in large cities and, for example, the major health effects of the world's largest ship breaking industry in Gujarat are front page issues. The District health authorities interviewed did not consider these occupational and environmental health issues as their prime responsibility, despite the fact that such interventions may be more cost effective than additional investments in clinical medical health services'. (EU 2007)

Bossert and Beauvais (2002) reported similar findings in Uganda, where decentralization actually increased the proportion of local spending allocated to hospitals and curative services and reduced public health interventions and primary health care.

The lesson from these experiences is that whatever administrative system is established, if the organisations are controlled by medical professionals or if the medical professionals have the greater share of the power, their preferences will determine what services are provided and how. The 'clan' mode of governance, through which professional ethics, standards, preferences and training determine the professionals' behaviour, produces outcomes that reflect the professions.

The moves away from clan governance, either towards hierarchy or market, have been made in part with the intention of changing the services to reflect other values.

Decentralising Through the Market

The creation of real or quasi-markets in health systems has been attempted in several jurisdictions as part of the reform process. The use of contracts that emulate market transactions or that are market transactions can be seen as a way of solving a 'principal–agent' problem, the Ministry of Health or similar being the principal and the other players in the system being treated as agents. One example of this sort of contract is the UK from 1997 to 2010, where there were Public Service Agreements for all public services, cascading down from the Treasury (the UK name for the Ministry of Finance) through departments to service delivery units. In the health case, the targets were set for the Strategic Health Authorities, through the Primary Care Trusts, responsible for commissioning services and down through the contracts with public and private providers of services. The system was monitored through two regulatory bodies, the Care Quality Commission and Monitor (Flynn 2012, pp. 130–134). The control mechanisms and where contracting fits in the process is illustrated in Fig. 4.1:

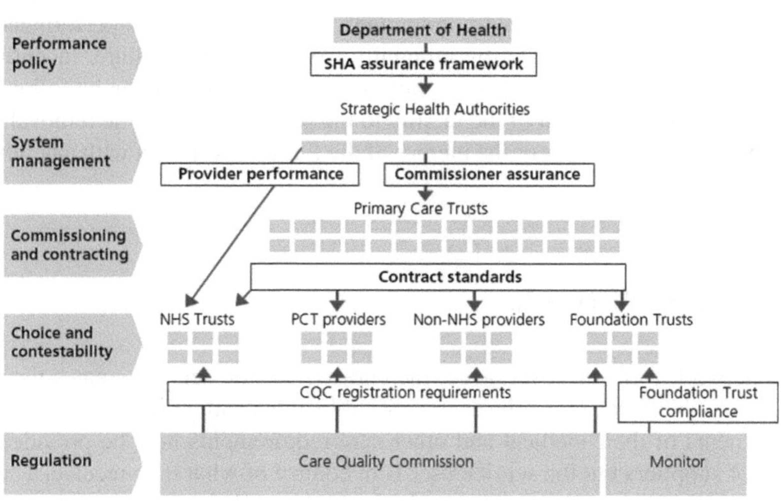

Fig. 4.1 Components of decentralization. Source: NHS (2008)

A second example is the cascade of agreements for primary care in Bolivia from national level to mid-level institutions to municipalities (Mitchell and Bossert 2010, p. 687). In this case the standards are expressed as health outcomes and the lower levels of administration are required to devise their own strategies to meet those standards. In both cases, the governance mechanism is a contractual arrangement that focuses accountability up the hierarchical chain, and in both cases there were in addition measures to focus accountability downwards to service users and local citizens.

The other purpose of markets and quasi-markets as a governance mechanism is to introduce competition as a way of reducing cost and improving quality, on the premise that behaviours in markets are superior for outcomes than behaviours in other governance systems. In the UK case the commissioning bodies have a series of contracts with service providers, both long-term block contracts and shorter term spot contracts, based on procedures followed. These contracts can be with state-owned service providers and private providers, either for profit or not for profit. Generally prices are pre-set and the competition is organised on the basis of available capacity or quality.

Use of the market as a governance mechanism, relies on the existence of a conducive market structure. In densely populated areas with a variety of service providers, competition may result in improved standards and a general attention to costs of service. In less densely populated places, there is likely to be a monopoly of provision, at least for more specialised services. The success of decentralization through the market depends on the degree of competition, the capacity of the competing units to manage in response to the competitive environment and the consequences of success or failure. The capacity to respond to the market depends on the degree to which control over human resources and other assets is devolved to the managers: competition with fixed salary levels and central controls on procurement and investment is unlikely to improve performance. The consequences of success and failure entail the incentives for individuals' and organisational performances. If a service provider is protected by immunity from closure or failure, incentives to perform are reduced. In the UK case, failure of a state provider can be followed by the transfer of management of the facility to the private sector or the removal of the local board by the Minister or the merger of the failing institution with a neighbouring successful one.

Decentralised Networks

In the network form of governance, the end user of the service creates their own network of which they are at the centre, possibly aided and guided by professionals. The elements of their medical and other care requirements may be provided by a variety of suppliers but the service user is in control of what they receive. The pure form is very rare, except for rich people. In insurance-based systems, the provider of the insurance will normally set criteria of eligibility and nominate acceptable service providers. In state-funded systems rationing criteria are in place to limit eligibility and access.

However, the network mode of governance, with the service user as 'customer' with the rights that come with being a customer is an ideal type based on neo-liberal principles. There have been a series of experiments in the UK to enable patients to 'choose and book' their service, through the medium of a general practitioner. For people needing social services inputs, there have also been regimes of personal budgets through which people purchase their chosen care, after meeting general eligibility criteria.

In principle, this form of governance puts the patient at the centre and makes the service providers compete for their business. The difference between governance through the market, as described above, and governance through a citizen-centred network is the role of the individual citizen or service user.

The gap in the health systems that are left by the network approach is the provision of public health services, which are essentially public goods. The attention to individual needs and preferences leads to a focus on curative interventions and way from preventive measures and matters such as water supply and quality, sanitation and food hygiene.

By definition, the provision of public goods is not best done either through the market or through a consumer-centred network mode of governance. The non-excludability of the benefits public health measures implies an alternative governance mode for successful policy outcomes.

'Good Governance'

This chapter has used a formal definition of governance that is narrower than that currently used by international agencies. The World Bank, for example, in 2011 defined governance in a much broader way:

> 'We define governance as the traditions and institutions by which authority in a country is exercised for the common good. This includes (I) the process by which those in authority are selected, monitored and replaced, (II) the capacity of government to effectively manage its resources and implement sound policies, and (III) the respect of citizens and the state for the institutions that govern economic and social interactions among them'. (p. 41)

This definition is endorsed by the World Health Organisation (2012) and is included in its definition of good governance for health. The WHO also supports the UNDP's (1997) even broader definition that states that the elements of good governance include accountability, transparency, responsiveness, equity and inclusiveness, effectiveness and efficiency, adherence to the rule of law, participation and consensus orientation.

These broad definitions of governance arise from the decision that the International Financial Institutions and the United Nations agencies should not interfere or make loan conditions about political matters which are subject to national sovereignty. They allow the agencies to comment and steer matters which would normally be considered part of politics by relabeling them as governance. 'How those in authority are selected', for example, and equity and inclusiveness are features of political systems. Rothstein (2012) has pointed out that the definition of 'good' governance cannot be restricted to a particular set of institutional arrangements, since many forms of government create good governance. Rather, he offers impartiality in the exercise of public power as the essence of good governance: 'Such a definition of *good governance* would make it clear what the norm is—that is, what is being "abused" when corruption, clientilism, favouritism, patronage, nepotism, or undue support to special interest groups occurs when a society is governed in a manner that should be considered as "good"' (p.152).

The relationship between decentralization and these broad definitions of governance, or good governance, is ambiguous. The first element of the World Bank definition, 'the process by which those in authority are selected', is neutral in respect to decentralization: boards of sub-national health bodies can be appointed by Ministers or elected by local people. Similarly the capacity at local level may be effective or ineffective, and citizens may or may not respect local institutions as much as they respect national ones. With regard to corruption, there are probably as many cases of theft and bribery at local as national levels of health systems.

The formal systems of allocation of responsibilities among national, intermediate and local levels are insufficient to ensure 'good' governance. What is required is governance mechanisms at whatever level to ensure behaviours that generate performance and accountability. Using Rothenberg's definition, we should ask whether there are processes and structures in place to ensure impartiality in a decentralised system. By definition decentralization implies local discretion: if that discretion is extended to include the choice of service recipient, then all of Rothstein's potential abuses may occur at local level.

Case Examples

Case Study: Spain (Extracted from Duran 2011)

'The Ministry of Health and Inter-territorial Council have encountered serious obstacles to effectively coordinating health and (especially) health service policies due to partisan struggles between national and regional political parties. As a result, geographical differences in health outcomes and financing as well as intraregion inequities arguably have changed little; average life expectancy at birth for both sexes ranges from 82.5 in Navarra to 79.8 in Andalucia. Since differences in health status reflect income and wealth differences, it would be unfair to blame the health system decentralization process entirely, yet as pointed out by Montero-Granados et al 'healthcare decentralization in Spain seems to show no positive effect on convergence in health, as measured

(continued)

by life expectancy at birth and infant mortality between provinces... Some provinces improved their situation overtaking others but the final result is one of greater dispersion than at the start". The real issue is that decentralization has kept per capita expenditure uneven. The SNS ['Sistema Nacional de Salud'—National Health System] Cohesion and Quality Law (2003) created the National Cohesion Fund to promote policies addressing geographic inequalities but it has primarily been used to pay for costs generated by patients being treated in health care facilities in regions other than their own, failing to promote the expected degree of national cohesion and reductions in inequality.

Furthermore, in the period 1992–2009 the variation coefficient of expenses among regions increased—and changes in population-protected volume fail to explain such variability. Legislation was passed in December 2009 to create a new regional financial system around a Guarantee Fund for Fundamental Public Services which integrated the Cohesion Fund, and holds 80 % of the resources for key public services such as education, social services and health care. Monies for the Fund are collected centrally from tax revenues and then dispersed. However, critics argue that arrangements disproportionately reflect the demands of some regions (namely Cataluña) in the context of electoral politics. Publicly funded health care expenses (budgeted) per person in 2010 still differed by (ie. 40.73 % of the average of Euro1343) between the Balearic Islands (79.37 % of the average) and the Basque Country (120.84 %). There is little wonder then that the Spanish health care system shows unwarranted variability in access, quality, safety and efficiency, across regions, health care areas and hospitals, including:

- 5-fold variation in the use of percutaneous transluminal coronary angioplasty (PTCA) between areas and 2-fold variation in mortality after PTCA (hospitals)
- 7.7-fold variability in prostatectomy rates across health care areas
- 28 times more frequent admissions to acute care hospitals due to affective psychosis between health areas;—26 % of hospitals with between 501 and 1,000 beds are at least 15 % more inefficient than the average
- 12 % of hospitals with between 201and 500 beds are at least 25 % less efficient than the standard for treating similar patients

Remarkably, the population does seem to perceive the lack of geographical equity in financing: only 42 % of respondents in the *Health Barometer* survey believe that the same health services are offered to all citizens despite region of residence, compared with around 87 % who assess treatment is equal despite patient's gender and around 70 % who assess treatment is equal despite a patient's social class and wealth' (p. 11).

Case Study: Poland (Extracted from Rincker and Battle 2011)

Despite stories of successful decentralization, there are also negative outcomes of decentralization. These include inadequate capacity of some provincial administrators and 'political meddling' in Patient Fund contracting which made the system as inefficient and political as the one it replaced. National or regional officials, with little reason to support budgets being given to Patient Fund directors, could intervene in Patient Fund politics and often tried to ensure that important providers or hospitals be given government contracts. In an interview, a Patient Fund employee described how provincial political ties determined health care contracts rather than concern for efficiency:

> There was a rural *powiat* [county] hospital outside of Limowa that was very badly in debt, and going to be liquidated. This public hospital was in danger of closing, and there were problems with the unions. The hospital building had been given to it by the county government. Then the *powiat* decided to rent out the property to a private owner. The owner of the private hospital was a member of the local government. After three years the hospital became private, but now the *powiat* official says he cannot rent out the building to a private hospital. So, a well-running private hospital will probably be closed to protect a public county hospital. The hospital will be re-publicized as an outlying department by the *powiat* leader, who essentially paid money to himself. There was pressure from the hospital director and unions to protect the public hospital.

This example of health care services under Poland's health decentralization system shows that incentives for politicians to reward connections and public entities can undermine efforts to make decentralised systems competitive and transparent and reduce public support for decentralization. In this example, it is notable that *powiat* officials who choose to reward friends with political connections over efficient health providers should be removed through the electoral process, but the problem of citizen awareness and accountability may persist in provincial- or lower-level politics as well as in national politics (p. 348).

Case Study Indonesia (Extracted from Simatupang 2009)

'…decentralization does not bring improvement in health service delivery for most municipalities in Indonesia. There is strong significant improvement for majority of municipalities in mortality related measures such as Under 5 Mortality Rate and life expectancy at birth, but most municipalities experience declining usage of health facilities (physical facilities and personnel). Indicators such as health service utilization rate, labor attended by medical workers, immunization coverage and contraceptive usage are worsen in most

(continued)

municipalities after decentralization. The results are contradictory; since improvements in mortality-related measures indicate better health care in general but service utilization measures are worsen after decentralization.

One possible explanation for the contradictory results in health service delivery is the uneven distribution of health services. While not all municipalities could build their own hospital, but there should be more community health clinics (*Puskesmas*), ancillary health clinic or mobile clinic available at the municipal level. It is likely that decentralization does not improve the distribution of health services, which people have to travel to the neighboring districts to enjoy health care service. These results express the need of health service reform in Indonesia to improve access to health services.

The uneven distribution of health services is more visible when we examine the determinants of changes in health outcomes. Result shows that after decentralization, the municipalities that already enjoy higher health services (i.e., have higher average number of health centers and health workers) allocate more resources to health sector compared to those municipalities that presently lacking of health services. Another measure of local needs, average number of epidemic occurred within a year, does not have statistically significant effect to health outcomes.

Similar to the results to education sector, the presence of civic, social institutions and private sector are positively related to health outcomes. Municipalities with more social organizations have higher service utilization rate, vaccination coverage and contraception usage, while active private sector economy lead to lower mortality measures. Results show that some health indicators are positively related with fiscal capacity. This indicates that municipalities with higher fiscal capacity increase their health expenditure, thus contributing to better service provision and better health outcomes. However, this add to unequal distribution in health service, as richer municipalities (i.e. higher own source revenue) will have much better health service than the poorer municipalities while municipalities with lower fiscal capacity (and less health service) will enjoy positive externality provided by their richer neighbors' (pp. 86–87).

Conclusions

The policy of decentralising health care operates within an existing governance system. From a historical institutional perspective, we would expect that the existing relationships will have an impact on the newly created relationships that result from the decentralization.

What we have seen from the examples is that a hierarchy can reassert itself even when policy makers' intentions have been to devolve power down a hierarchy. Those whose power is threatened by the new relationships will use whatever means they can to retain their control. This may be through funding mechanisms, through HR systems or by control over central aspects of the policy process. The requirement, for example, to provide 'core' services will reduce the autonomy of local governance units.

An extreme version of the maintenance of the hierarchy is seen in the contractual approach through which the centre asserts itself as the 'principal' and the devolved or local units are treated as if they are 'agents' of the centre. This is achieved through the contractual means of attaching output conditions to the flow of funds from the centre to the devolved units.

Clan control generally operates through the maintenance of values irrespective of the formal, official governance mechanisms. Medical staff may not alter their behaviours because of the existence of formal, hierarchical command and control processes. Plans, budgets, targets and performance management systems all require conformance from those delivering services. Ethical stances and professional preferences can undermine such mechanisms and reassert professional standards and therefore behaviours.

Decentralization when governance operates though the market will be subject to all the constraints identified by institutional economics, especially market structure and the distribution of information among the players in the market. Decentralization does not automatically produce the welfare gains identified by Musgrave. Decentralization policy is mediated through governance mechanisms, and those mechanisms have an impact on outcomes, whether the overall control of the system is centralised or decentralised. In any case, centralisation may be more likely to produce two of the desired outcomes of a health care system: productive efficiency and equitable distribution of health care. Decentralization is capable of supporting corruption as well as responsiveness and local accountability.

Discussion Topics

1. Is it inevitable that decentralised governance for health care reduces the equity of access to care and health outcomes among the areas to which control is devolved? What would national governments have to do to ensure equity? And would these measures inevitably produce re-centralisation?
2. What are the factors that create a tendency towards central control, even when governments intend to decentralise health care governance?
3. Does 'clan' governance undermine attempts to manage health care provision?
4. Does decentralization inevitably lead to more corruption, nepotism and patrimonialism in health care? What needs to be done to ensure impartiality within health care systems at local level?

Case Study Questions

Indonesia: What is the explanation for increased inequality of health service access after decentralization of health care?

What else could be done to reduce inequality of access?

Poland: In the example of the hospital that was transferred to the private ownership of a member of the local authority, what changes to governance would be necessary to prevent a repeat of such an action?

Spain: Is it inevitable that political decentralization will result in disparities in health care provision and health outcomes?

Recommended Reading

Saltman, R. B., Bankausskaite, V., & Frangbæk, K. (2007). *Decentralization in health care.* Maidenhead: Open University Press/McGraw Hill.

A comprehensive survey of approaches to and results of decentralization in health care.

References

Bossert, T. J., & Beauvais, J. C. (2002). Decentralization of health systems in Ghana, Zambia, Uganda and the Philippines: A comparative analysis of decision space. *Health Policy and Planning, 17*(1), 14–31.

Cassels, A. (1995). Health sector reform: Key issues in less developed countries. *Journal of International Development, 7*(3), 329–347.

Durán, A. (2011). Health system decentralization in Spain: A complex balance, Euro Observer. *The Health Policy Bulletin, 13*(1).

European Union, (2007, August). *Evaluation of European Commission's Support to the Republic of India*, Final Report.

Flynn, N. (2012). *Public sector management.* London: Sage.

Mitchell, A., & Bossert, T. (2010). Decentralization: Governance and health-system performance: 'Where You Stand Depends on Where You Sit'. *Development Policy Review, 28*(6), 669–691.

Musgrave, R. A. (1959). *The theory of public finance.* New York: McGraw Hill.

National Health Service UK (2008), *'Developing the NHS Performance Regime'*

Rincker, M., & Battle, M. (2011). Dissatisfied with decentralization: Explaining citizens' evaluations of Poland's 1999 Health Care Reforms. *Perspectives on European Politics and Society, 12*(3), 340–357.

Rondinelli, A. (1983). *Decentralization in developing countries.* Work Bank Staff Working paper 581

Rothstein, B. (2012). Good governance. In D. Levi-Faur (Ed.), *Oxford handbook of governance.* Oxford: OUP.

Saltman, R. B., Bankausskaite V., & Frangbæk, K. (2007). *Decentralization in health care.* Open University Press/McGraw Hill.

Simatupang, R. R. (2009). *Evaluation of decentralization outcomes in Indonesia: Analysis of health and education sectors.* Economics Dissertation, Georgia State University

UNDP, (1997). *Good governance and sustainable human development.* New York United Nations Development Programme.

Williamson, O. (1975). *Markets and hierarchies: Analysis and anti-trust implications*. New York: Free Press.

World Bank. (2011). *What is our approach to governance?* Washington: Word Bank.

World Health Organisation, (2012). *Governance for health in the 21*st *century*, WHO Regional Office for Europe.

Chapter 5
Fiscal Decentralization of Health Services

Dolores Jiménez-Rubio

Abstract This chapter presents the main economic arguments for and against devolution in the allocation of public expenses and revenues to subnational governments. It then explores the implications that follow from fiscal decentralization to the health sector in particular. The most common indicators of fiscal decentralization used in the research literature are discussed, together with their benefits and limitations. The chapter concludes by providing a summary of the current empirical evidence on the relationship between different measures of fiscal decentralization and various health outcome indicators.

After Reading This Chapter You Will Be Able to

- *Identify the key theoretical strengths and weaknesses associated with fiscal decentralization of health services.*
- *Distinguish among the various intergovernmental arrangements that may exist in devolved health-care systems.*
- *Understand the existing evidence on the effect of the fiscal dimension of decentralization on health care as well as the ways forward in this area.*

Activity 1

What is the main purpose of intergovernmental grants? What are the problems associated with an excessive reliance of grants on the part of sub national governments?

D. Jiménez-Rubio (✉)
Department of Applied Economics, University of Granada, Campus de Cartuja S/N, Granada 18071, Spain
e-mail: dolores@ugr.es

K. Regmi (ed.), *Decentralizing Health Services: A Global Perspective*,
DOI 10.1007/978-1-4614-9071-5_5,

Effect of Fiscal Decentralization on Health Services: Challenges and Opportunities

In recent years many countries have moved towards more decentralization of their health-care systems. In the UK, the Scottish and Welsh Assemblies were created in 1999 providing limited discretion to Scotland and Wales over health services, among other policies. And there is a continuing debate about the need for increasing the financial accountability of both the Scottish and Welsh Assemblies, in the sense of making them more accountable for their sources of revenue. Also, in traditionally more decentralised countries such as Spain or Italy, regional governments have also seen recently increased their responsibility over their sources of revenue.

While decentralization is very often politically motivated, it can have important effects on economic issues such as efficiency in the provision of public services, equity and economic growth. The beneficial impact of decentralization is based on the assumptions that decentralization can improve the information of local decision makers about local circumstances, stimulating prompt and effective responses to local needs, and is an effective channel for people to express their preferences making local decision makers more accountable to local citizens' demands (Oates 1999). Local decision makers also have more opportunities to reduce costs than central managers. They can tailor staff and procedures to the local context and have more freedom for experimenting with alternative ways of doing things and implementing them rather than relying on centrally determined procedures. Therefore, decentralization, if properly designed and implemented, is expected to improve equity, efficiency, quality, access to health-care services, and ultimately health outcomes.

Successful implementation of decentralization requires a complex balance between political, fiscal and administrative policies. All of these elements should complement each other if the aim is to deliver public services of quality and strengthen fiscal discipline and responsiveness of local governments (something which has been labelled as the "Soufflé Theory"). In order to promote responsiveness of policymakers for the provision of public services and efficiency in the management of economic resources, decentralization should encompass a clear division of responsibilities and a transparent system of accountability (World Bank 2013a). While intergovernmental fiscal transfers may be required on equity grounds to compensate for different revenue capacities at the local level, there is a risk that too much reliance on grants places little pressure on local governments to reduce costs (Oates 1993). This is because by breaking the links between the costs and benefits, transfers make it difficult for voters to identify and penalise the causes of local inefficiencies in the use of resources (Rodden 2003). In the health-care sector in particular, there is some evidence suggesting that health-care spending by subnational governments is not responsive to reductions in transfers from the central government, implying that regions prefer to incur in deficits than to reducing health-care expenditure (Levaggi and Zanola 2003).

Potential gains to be realised from decentralization are also conditional on the existence of decentralization of political decision-making authority, and, in particular, effective channels for the individuals to express their preferences, and incentives for the policymakers to respond to those preferences. For this reason many authors are sceptical about the successful implementation of decentralization in less developing countries, given their weaker administrative capacity and their lower initial levels of democracy as compared to developed countries (Khaleghian 2004; Bossert and Mitchell 2011). Previous studies have shown that some of the consequences of institutional environments with weak political rights and governance include low local expertise in management, poor accountability and local participation, elite capture and limited fiscal resources, all of which translate in a reduction in the efficiency in the allocation of resources. These effects might undermine the desirable impact of decentralization on health outcomes.

In spite of the compelling theoretical arguments put forward for devolution of policymaking, and health services in particular, decentralization is not without its limitations (Khaleghian 2004; Costa-i-Font 2012a). Regarding economies of scale, decentralization might generate inefficient location of facilities such as hospitals by local decision makers accountable to local electors. Central intervention in health care is also expected to result in more efficient pricing of inputs by a single purchaser of health care. Decentralization of health services with important externalities, such as immunisation services, is expected to encourage local jurisdictions to "free-ride" on the immunisation status of their neighbours. The result could be a suboptimal disease protection level provided in the country as a whole. Finally, unless the central government coordinates an adequate transfer mechanism from richer to poorer regions, decentralization may result in increased inequalities in health care if local authorities under pressures to raise their own revenues rely on user fees to finance their services or reduce the coverage of the universal health package.

Inequality in health outcomes (e.g. Montero-Granados et al. 2007) or in the access to health services following decentralization can also be considered as a natural and not necessarily negative consequence of this policy but rather as a reflection of the different regional priorities according to its preferences and needs. Some authors go even further and argue that inequalities could be regarded as a challenge for inefficient regions to perform better if a system of political incentives is in place and information about the outcomes of the system is freely available (Costa-i-Font 2012b). The most appropriate level of decentralization of health services is therefore a key policy issue that to date remains largely unresolved.

Characterising the Fiscal Dimension of Decentralization

The level of decentralization in policymaking is a complex phenomenon embracing a number of political, fiscal and administrative dimensions. As we have seen in the previous section, all these elements should complement each other in order to deliver public services of quality and increase fiscal discipline and accountability of local governments. Therefore, an accurate measure of decentralization should be able to capture a wide variety of issues such as political autonomy (range of services

Table 5.1 Describing the level of fiscal autonomy of subnational governments

Share of subnational spending on total spending
Share of government revenue raised and retained by subnational governments
Share of "shared revenue" in subnational spending/revenue
Percentage of local expenditures funded through local revenues
Percentage of local expenditures funded through intergovernmental transfers
Percentage of local expenditures funded through local revenues
Discretion in allocating expenditure across and within sectors

Source: Decentralization Toolkit, World Bank (2013a)

to be covered or access conditions in the health sector) or the legal and regulatory structure (e.g. service standards, training regulations). The crucial aspect is whether the key features of public policy and the health-care system in particular are defined centrally or whether there is substantial scope for regional variation and for subnational government's involvement in defining the basic rules of the system (Banting and Corbett 2002). However, since many of these considerations are not easy to measure empirically, in the absence of more appropriate data, only the fiscal dimension has been traditionally used to characterise decentralization in the research literature following Oates' seminal work in 1972. Table 5.1 summarises some of the main features which characterise discretion of local governments in the management of economic resources according to the World Bank (2013a).

The most commonly used dataset to generate measures of fiscal decentralization is the International Monetary Fund's (IMF) Government Finance Statistics (GFS). GFS data distinguishes between the spending and revenue patterns of central, state and local governments, thereby providing useful information for the purpose of analysing decentralization. GFS-based decentralization indicators typically measure the share of subnational (state and local) spending or revenue in the total spending or revenue for all levels of government (central, state and local). GFS also offers relevant information on vertical imbalances, that is, the degree to which subnational governments rely on transfers to finance their expenditures. In addition, for some countries government expenditure can be further classified into health and education. This is an important strength of GFS data for studying decentralization in health services in particular, since countries can vary in the way they assign their expenditure responsibilities to local governments.

Figure 5.1 shows that in some countries such as Romania, the Netherlands or Iceland, subnational governments are responsible for spending around a quarter of the total spending of all layers of government. However, health-care spending seems to be directly controlled and managed by the central government. By contrast, in countries such as Denmark, South Africa or Spain, expenditures for health-care services are highly decentralised relative to other sectors, in the sense that health-care spending is mostly spent by regional authorities. Only in some countries such as Mauritius, the USA or Norway, overall fiscal decentralization appears to represent well the level of decentralization in the health services. Therefore, using overall fiscal decentralization indicators to proxy the level of decentralization in health care

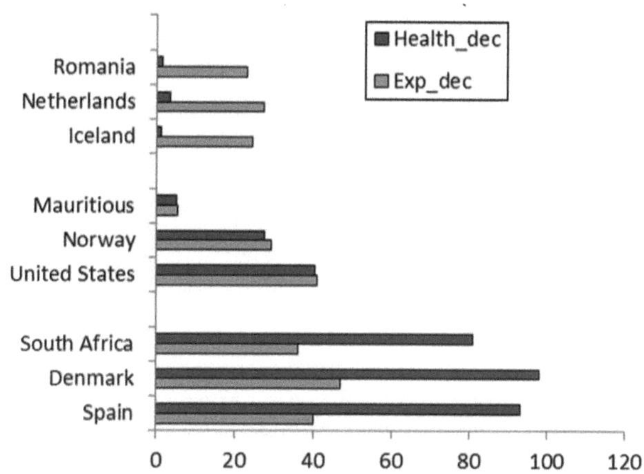

Fig. 5.1 Sub national government share of expenditure vs sub national government share of health expenditure in selected countries. 2010[ab]. Source: Own elaboration from World Bank Fiscal Decentralization dataset (2013b)

[a] Data for 2010 or latest available year

[b]Health decentralization (Health_dec) denotes the proportion of local and state expenditures on health over the total (central, state and local). Expenditure decentralization (Exp_dec) denotes the proportion of total expenditures accounted for by sub national (state or local) governments.

would result in an overestimation in the case of Romania, the Netherlands and Iceland and an underestimation in Spain, Denmark and South Africa.

While providing a consistent dataset across countries and over time, decentralization measures based on data from the GFS are not without their limitations. First of all, GFS data may provide a misleading picture of the real level of autonomy in policymaking of subnational tiers of government (Ebel and Yilmaz 2002; Rodden 2003). This is because GFS's local spending statistics include not only expenditures controlled totally or partially by local jurisdictions but also expenditures in functions controlled by higher levels of government through directives or earmarked grants, that is, grants which can only be used for specific purposes. By contrast, non-earmarked grants provide local governments with the flexibility to spend the money as if it were subnational government's own revenue. On the other hand, the GFS classifies revenues which give local governments little tax autonomy as subnational own-source revenue. These include "shared taxes", which are effectively another form of an intergovernmental transfer, and taxes which allow local authorities to set the tax rate and/or base. As a consequence, both revenue- and expenditure-based GFS data may overestimate the true level of decentralization.

In recent years the OECD has substantially improved the fiscal information available for a selected group of OECD countries by classifying taxes according to the level of discretion entitled to their local governments. This classification ranges from (a.) where the central government can set both the rate of taxation and the tax base to (e.) where subnational governments set both the tax base and the tax rate. Tax sharing agreements are further arranged into four categories from (d.1.) where the subnational governments can determine the revenue split to (d.4.) where the

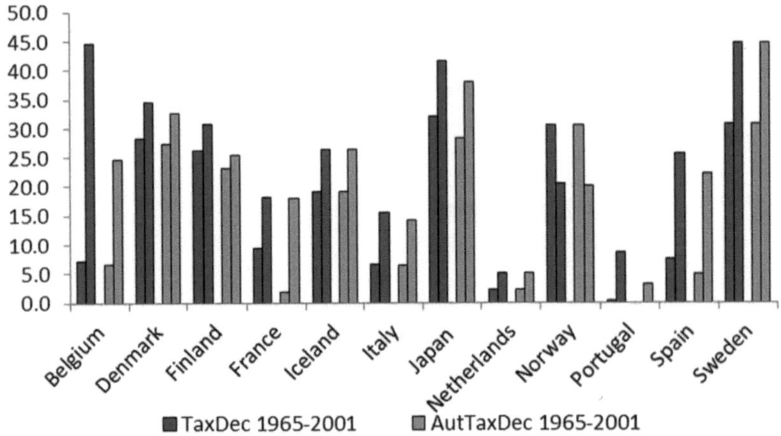

Fig. 5.2 Evolution of fiscal decentralization measures: countries with an upwards trend. 1965-2001[ab]. Source: Own elaboration from Stegarescu's dataset (2005)
[a] Fiscal data for 1965 or earliest available year and 2001 or latest available year
[b] Tax decentralization (TaxDec) denotes the sub national tax revenue over general government total revenue (central, state and local). Autonomous tax decentralization (AutTaxDec) denotes the share ofsub national tax revenue over the total revenue but only includes those taxes where the sub national government can change the tax rate, the tax base or both

national government can unilaterally determine the revenue split. Moreover, the OECD reports annual data on the type of intergovernmental transfers ("conditional" versus "earmarked") in a selected sample of countries since year 2000. While this data offers interesting new perspectives on the intergovernmental arrangements of these countries, it is somewhat limited to empirically assess the effect of fiscal decentralization since the tax autonomy information is only collected for selected years (1995, 2002, 2008 and 2010).

Drawing on the OECD classification of taxing powers of subnational governments, Stegarescu (2005) extended the OECD dataset to cover 23 countries from 1965 to 2001. Fiscal decentralization therefore measures the share of local government taxes over the general government but only considers those taxes where the local government has powers over the tax rate, the tax base or both. This dataset represents a major improvement for evaluating the effects of fiscal decentralization compared to conventional indicators of decentralization based on IMF GFS data.

According to Figs. 5.2 and 5.3, there are many countries where all taxes allocated to local governments are autonomous (Austria, Canada, Iceland, Luxembourg, the Netherlands, New Zealand, Norway, Sweden, the UK, the USA). In some other countries, however, only a small proportion of the local taxes provide local governments with the power to control the tax rate and/or the tax base. These include Australia, Germany and, to a lower extent, Portugal.

The evolution of autonomous tax and total tax decentralization shows a similar trend over the period studied with only two exceptions. These are Australia, where autonomous tax decentralization (AutTaxDec) slightly increases over the period of

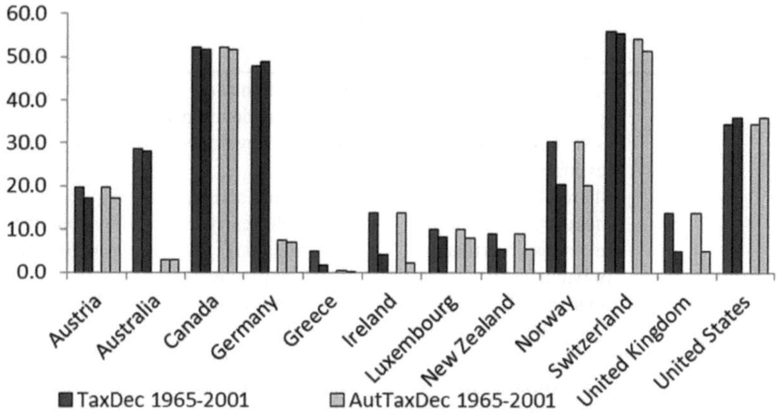

Fig. 5.3 Evolution of fiscal decentralization measures: countries with a stable or a downwards trend.1965-2001[ab]. Source: Own elaboration from Stegarescu's dataset (2005)
[a] Fiscal data for- 1965 or earliest available year and 2001 or latest available year
[b] Tax decentralization (TaxDec) denotes the sub national tax revenue over general government total revenue (central, state and local). Autonomous tax decentralization (AutTaxDec) denotes the share of sub

study, while total tax decentralization decreases (TaxDec), and Germany, where the opposite holds (see Fig. 5.3).

With respect to AutTaxDec, the improved measure of fiscal decentralization, a trend towards increasing fiscal powers of subnational governments over the period 1965–2001 can be observed in many countries but especially in Belgium, Italy and Spain (see Fig. 5.3). Ireland, New Zealand, Norway and the UK have experienced a reduction in the level of subnational fiscal autonomy, while the remaining countries, which are traditional federal countries, have shown a fairly stable degree of fiscal decentralization over the period of study (see Fig. 5.2). According to Stegarescu (2005), AutTaxDec is a reliable indicator that reflects well the institutional changes that have taken place in these countries over the 30 years of study.

To conclude, despite its limitations, to date IMF GFS data offers the most comprehensive source of information on intergovernmental fiscal relations. Treated with caution, GFS-based fiscal measures can provide useful insights on the evolution of decentralization of economic resources across time and among countries (see Table 5.2 for a summary of the decentralization indicators reviewed in this section).

Finally, there are several aspects that should be taken into account when measuring decentralization. First of all, indicators of fiscal decentralization conventionally employed in the literature do not capture important dimensions of the decentralization process such as political accountability and responsiveness to local needs. Second, some countries implement asymmetric, gradual processes of devolution of policy-making to subnational governments. This is the case of Spain where the process of decentralization of health services to regions spread over a period of 20 years starting in 1981. In these circumstances the use of aggregate data could be misleading, whereas

Table 5.2 Summary of main fiscal decentralization indicators[a]

Source	Decentralization variables	Strengths	Weaknesses
IMF GFS fiscal data	–SN share of government spending/revenue in total government spending/revenue –Share of intergovernmental transfers in SN revenues ("vertical imbalances") –Share of SN own revenues	–Comprehensive coverage: developed and less developed countries –Long time series available (early seventies on) –Health-specific information for expenditure-based decentralization	–Unbalanced dataset –Data does not reveal real level of autonomy in expenditure/revenue of SN governments
OECD Fiscal Decentralization Indicators	–Proportion of SN "autonomous" own tax revenues –Share of grants revenue of SN governments by type of grant	–Distinguishes by type of grant (earmarked versus non-earmarked) and classifies taxes according to autonomy of SN governments	–Unbalanced dataset –For taxes, coverage only for selected years (1995, 2002, 2008, 2010)
Stegarescu's fiscal autonomy measures	–Proportion of SN "autonomous" own tax revenues	–Classifies taxes according to the taxing power of SN authorities –Long times series (1965–2001)	–Unbalanced dataset –Data not up to date (it does not go beyond 2001)

[a]*SN* stands for subnational

the use of country-specific comparisons of decentralised versus non-decentralised samples provides an optimal approach for evaluating the effect of decentralization. Third, studies of fiscal decentralization should make a clear distinction between developed and less developed countries since the allocation of public resources tends to differ among the two (for instance, in poorer countries local authorities tend to rely more on taxes collected by the central government such as trade taxes).

Activity 2

What are the economic and political factors that should be considered when analyzing fiscal decentralization in less developed countries versus developed ones? In what ways could foreign aid undermine the potential benefits from decentralization?

On the foreign aid issue, see: Prud'homme "The Dangers of Decentralization 20 years later", World Bank, 2013. http://siteresources.worldbank.org/PUBLICSECTORANDGOVERNANCE/Resources/285741-1326399585993/8366509-1348151550697/DangersOfDecentralization.pdf.

Case Study 1

Table 5.1 summarizes the main aspects which according to the World Bank Decentralization Toolkit characterize the level of fiscal decentralization of a country. In practice, however, the fiscal and intergovernmental arrangements of countries can be very different making it difficult to assess the exact degree of autonomy in decision making. Use the World Bank and the OECD Fiscal Decentralization Databases to analyze and compare the level of fiscal policy making autonomy of the following countries: Canada, Spain and Sweden. These three OECD countries have in common highly decentralized health care sectors, but differ in the way they finance their expenditures and in the freedom that their sub national governments have over their own taxes. Are there similarities in any of their fiscal features (tax revenue autonomy, share of sub national health and total spending, etc)? What are the main differences that can be found among the three countries regarding fiscal decentralization? What are the key advantages and disadvantages of using each of the fiscal proxies for decentralization?

Empirical Evidence on the Effect of Fiscal Decentralization for Health Services

In recent years an increasing number of studies have investigated the impact of fiscal decentralization on various measures of population's health such as infant mortality, life expectancy or immunisation coverage rates. Table 5.3 summarises the main results of these studies. Overall, most of the literature finds a beneficial impact of decentralization on various measures of health.

Asfaw et al. (2007) show that decentralization has a positive influence on child mortality in Indian rural villages using an index of fiscal decentralization obtained by factor analysis on the basis of three fiscal decentralization variables for the period 1990–1997. The study by Habibi et al. (2003) shows that the percent of revenue raised locally and the proportion of controlled revenue over the total have a negative and significant association with infant mortality rates for a panel of Argentinean provinces over the period 1970–1994. In addition, the authors find that during the period of decentralization reforms studied, regional inequalities were considerably reduced. Using a panel data of low- and high-income countries, Robalino et al. (2001) find that a measure of expenditure decentralization is inversely related to infant mortality rates during the period 1970–1995. Interestingly, according to the results the marginal benefit from decentralization is greater at low-income levels.

In the study by Uchimura and Jütting (2009), two measures of fiscal decentralization of Chinese counties based on the counties' expenditures and revenues were found to be significantly associated with lower infant mortality between 1995 and

Table 5.3 Summary of previous literature on the impact of fiscal decentralization on health outcomes

Author	Area of study	Period of study	Fiscal decentralization variable	Main results
Asfaw et al. (2007)	Rural villages in India	1990–1997	Decentralization is proxied by an index of fiscal decentralization obtained by factor analysis on the basis of three variables (the share of local (rural) expenditure on total state (intermediate government tier) expenditure, the total local expenditure per rural population and the share of local own revenue from the total local expenditure)	This study suggests that fiscal decentralization is negatively related to infant mortality rates. Political decentralization is a potential factor that can affect the effectiveness of fiscal decentralization
Cantarero and Pascual (2008)	15 Spanish regions	1992–2003	The key indicator of decentralization is the ratio of subnational health-care expenditure to the total health expenditure for all the levels of government	Fiscal decentralization is found to be negatively related to infant mortality over the period of study
Habibi et al. (2003)	23 Argentinean provinces	1970–1994	Two key decentralization indicators: percentage of revenue raised locally and proportion of controlled revenue over the total	Decentralization has a negative and significant association with infant mortality rates. In addition, the study shows that during the period of decentralization reforms studied, inequalities between richer and poorer regions were considerably reduced
Jiménez-Rubio (2010)	Ten provinces of Canada	1979–1995	Ratio of provincial health-care expenditure over the total health expenditure for all levels of government	Decentralization appears to have a considerable effect in reducing infant mortality rates in Canadian provinces
Jiménez-Rubio (2011)	20 OECD countries	1970–2001	Proportion of local revenue over total government revenue and proportion of revenue over which local governments can determine the tax base, the tax rate or both	Only the proportion of local "autonomous" tax revenue is found to exert a significant effect in infant mortality

Khaleghian (2004)	140 low- and middle-income countries	1980–1997	Two indicators of fiscal decentralization were used: a.) binary variable defined as the presence of taxing, spending or regulatory authority on the part of subnational authorities and b.) a combination of two variables—the share of subnational expenditures on total government expenditures and the share of health spending on total subnational expenditures	Decentralization improves immunisation coverage rates only in low-income countries
Robalino et al. (2001)	Low- and high-income countries	1970–1995	Proportion of subnational government spending over central government spending	Decentralization is associated with lower infant mortality rates. The marginal benefit from decentralization is found to be greater at low-income levels
Soto et al. (2012)	1080 Colombian municipalities	1998–2007	Locally controlled health expenditure as a proportion of total health expenditure	The measure of fiscal decentralization is negatively related to infant mortality rate. However, the effect of decentralization appears to be stronger for richer regions
Uchimura and Jütting (2009)	26 Chinese provinces	1995–2001	The authors use a measure of the proportion of counties' expenditure financed by counties' revenue ("vertical balance") and the ratio of counties' aggregate expenditure to total provincial expenditure	The study finds that more decentralised provinces have lower infant mortality rates than more centralised ones if decentralization is funded primarily by counties' own sources of revenue

2001. Finally, the recent papers by Cantarero and Pascual (2008) and Jiménez-Rubio (2010) also find an inverse relationship between fiscal decentralization, measured as the ratio of subnational health-care spending over the total, and health outcomes in the Spanish regions and the Canadian provinces, respectively.

Two recent studies improve upon previous fiscal measures of decentralization by using indicators of the degree of discretion of subnational governments in managing their revenue and spending. Using Stegarescu's indicator of local taxing power for 20 OECD countries, Jiménez-Rubio (2011) shows that fiscal decentralization exerts a considerable positive effect on infant mortality over a 30-year time span (1970–2001) only if a considerable degree of autonomy in the sources of revenue is devolved to local governments. On the other hand, Soto et al. (2012) find that the rate of locally controlled health expenditures has a substantial effect in reducing infant mortality rate in Colombian municipalities in the period 1999–2007. The authors also show that, contrary to the results found by Robalino et al. (2001), on the basis of cross-country comparisons the magnitude of the effect appears to be stronger for richer regions.

Khaleghian (2004) examines the association between fiscal decentralization and an alternative health-related outcome: the coverage rates a key infant vaccine in 140 low- and middle-income countries during the period 1980–1997. Contrary to the expectations, the findings indicate that decentralization improves coverage rates only in low-income countries. The author explains this interesting result by the likely balance between responsiveness to local needs and the preservation of central influence necessary for the effective functioning of immunisation programmes in low-income countries.

Conclusion

This chapter introduced some of the main advantages and drawbacks that follow from the theory of fiscal federalism to the health services in particular. If well designed, decentralization can promote equity, efficiency, quality of service provision, access to health-care services and ultimately health outcomes. This requires, in addition to a strong system of political rights and liberties, a system of economic incentives in which local decision makers are held accountable for their spending decisions. The key features of a well-designed fiscal decentralization system were discussed in the second section of this chapter, along with the main databases which capture some of these dimensions. Finally, section three introduced the current evidence on the relationship between fiscal decentralization and health outcomes. These studies find in general a positive effect of decentralization on health-related outcomes. However, and in line with the theoretical literature, a number of studies show that an important condition for this to happen is that decentralization is funded primarily by economic resources which incentivise local decision makers to manage the spending in an efficient way.

While the growing volume of literature on fiscal decentralization has certainly informed the debate about the impact of this policy reform, current evidence on its benefits and costs to the health system is however limited by the following reasons. Firstly, by relying on fiscal data, much of the literature fails to capture other important aspects of decentralization in policymaking or the linkages between the various dimensions of decentralization. And secondly, there is a lack of evaluation of other aspects of the health-care system that may be influenced by fiscal decentralization such as its impact on the overall health-care costs to the system or equity in access to the system (if this is considered as a higher priority in a decentralised country than regional diversity on the basis of preferences or needs). Further research is therefore needed in order to establish firm conclusions about the merits of decentralising health services.

Case Study 2

Scotland will hold a referendum in 2014 to decide whether to be an independent, separate country, whether to get more devolved powers, or to maintain the "status quo". A commission to review and improve devolution produced a document summarized in The Economist in 2008 ("*An Attempt to make devolution work better creates as many problems as it solves*", 4 December, 2008).

- Could you describe the system proposed to increase devolution in Scotland?
- What would be the main advantages and disadvantages of this system?

Recommended Reading

Ahmad, E., & Brosio, G. (2006). *Handbook of fiscal federalism*. Washington DC: International Monetary Fund.

World Bank. Decentralization and Sub national Finance Website.

References

Asfaw, A., Frohberg, K., James, K. S., & Jütting, J. (2007). Fiscal decentralization and health outcomes: Empirical evidence from rural India. *Journal of Developing Areas, 41*, 17–35

Banting, K. G., & Corbett, S. (2002). *Health policy and federalism. A comparative perspective of multi-level governance*. Kingston: McGill-Queen's University Press.

Bossert, T., & Mitchell, A. (2011). Health sector decentralization and local-decision making: Decision space, institutional capacities and accountability in Pakistan. *Social Science and Medicine, 72*, 39–48.

Cantarero, D., & Pascual, M. (2008). Analysing the impact of fiscal decentralization on health outcomes: Empirical evidence from Spain. *Applied Economic Letters, 15*, 109–111.

Costa-i-Font, J. (2012a). Fiscal federalism and European health system decentralization: A perspective. LSE Europe in question discussion paper series, 55/2012. European Institute, London School of Economics and Political Science, London, UK.

Costa-i-Font, J. (2012b). Myths of health care decentralization. *Journal of Health Services Research and Policy, 17*(4), 252–253.

Ebel, R. D., & Yilmaz, S. (2002). *On the measurement and impact of fiscal decentralization. (World Bank Policy Research Working Paper No. 2809)*. Washington DC: World Bank.

Habibi, N., Huang, C., Miranda, D., Murillo, V., Ranis, G., Sarkar, M., et al. (2003). Decentralization and human development in Argentina. *Journal of Human Development, 4*(1), 73–101.

Jiménez-Rubio, D. (2010). Decentralization of health services and its impact on health outcomes: Evidence from Canada. *Applied Economics, 43*(26), 3907–3917.

Jiménez-Rubio, D. (2011). The impact of fiscal decentralization on infant mortality rates: Evidence from OECD countries. *Social Science and Medicine, 73*(9), 1401–1407.

Khaleghian, P. (2004). Decentralization and public services: The case of immunization. *Social Science and Medicine, 59*(1), 163–183.

Levaggi, R., & Zanola, R. (2003). Flypaper effect and sluggishness: Evidence from regional health expenditure in Italy. *International Tax and Public Finance, 10*, 535–547.

Montero-Granados, R., Jiménez-Aguilera, J. D., & Martín-Martín, J. J. (2007). Decentralization and convergence in health among the provinces of Spain (1980–2001). *Social Science and Medicine, 64*(6), 1253–1264.

Oates, W. E. (1993). Fiscal decentralization and economic development. *National Tax Journal, 46*(2), 237–243.

Oates, W. E. (1999). An essay on fiscal federalism. *Journal of Economic Literature, 37*, 1120–1149.

OECD. *OECD Fiscal Decentralization Database*. http://www.oecd.org/ctp/federalism/oecdfiscaldecentralizationdatabase.htm#A_1 Accessed 12 April 2013

Robalino, D. A., Picazo, O. F., & Voetberg, A. (2001). *Does fiscal decentralization improve health outcomes? Evidence from a cross-country analysis (Policy Research Working Paper No. 2565)*. Washington, DC: World Bank.

Rodden, J. (2003). Reviving Leviathan: Fiscal federalism and the growth of government. *International Organization, 57*, 695–729.

Soto, V. E., Farfan, M. I., & Lorant, V. (2012). Fiscal decentralization and infant mortality rate: The Colombian case. *Social Science and Medicine, 74*(9), 1426–1434.

Stegarescu, D. (2005). Public sector decentralization: Measurement concepts and recent international trends. *Fiscal Studies, 26*, 301–333.

Uchimura, H., & Jütting, J. (2009). Fiscal decentralization, Chinese style: Good for health outcomes? *World Development, 37*(12), 1924–1936.

World Bank (2013a). Decentralization toolkit. Decentralization and sub national Finance website.http://www1.worldbank.org/publicsector/decentralization/toolkit9.pdf Accessed 26 April 2013

World Bank (2013b). Fiscal decentralization indicators. Decentralization and sub national Finance website. http://siteresources.worldbank.org/PUBLICSECTORANDGOVERNANCE/Resources/285741-1326399585993/8366509-1332861347588/gfsDec2012_indicators_final.xlsx Accessed 11 March 2013

Chapter 6
Decentralized Planning Processes

Colin Thunhurst

Abstract In this chapter, we consider the essentials and the complexities of building decentralised planning systems. We will discuss critical issues such as the importance and the mechanisms for ensuring full community engagement. We will outline the importance of integrating planning systems across the different sectors and the difficulty of achieving decentralization within a single sector. We will present some practical tools, as well as considering overall structures. Throughout, although this aspect will not be explicitly addressed in this chapter, it will be clear that decentralization is an essentially political process, reflecting prevailing ideological perspectives on the appropriate distribution of power. In a subsequent chapter we will discuss the implications for information systems and the role of qualitative and quantitative measurement within health sectors.

After Reading This Chapter You Will be Able to

- *Understand the importance of implementing a decentralised health-care planning system to the achievement of the wider objectives of decentralization.*
- *Appreciate the specific features that are central to the successful implementation of a decentralised planning system.*
- *Recognise the different stages of the planning cycle and the respective outputs from those different stages.*

This chapter is dedicated to the memory of Carol Barker. Carol was to be co-author but died on 24 October 2012. Much of the ideas and work reported here were a result of the author's collaboration with Carol over a period of 25 years.

C. Thunhurst (✉)
Faculty of Health and Life Sciences, University of Coventry, Stone Cottage, 5 Aire View, Sandbeds, Keighley, West Yorkshire BD20 5LH, UK
e-mail: c.thunhurst@coventry.ac.uk

K. Regmi (ed.), *Decentralizing Health Services: A Global Perspective*,
DOI 10.1007/978-1-4614-9071-5_6, © Springer Science+Business Media New York 2014

- Appreciate the range of planning tools available and the specific contribution to the planning process of *problem structuring methods* and of the *logical framework approach.*

Introduction

Decentralised Planning

The purpose of decentralization is to move decision-making closer to the point at which decisions impact. This ensures that those decisions are more sensitive to their implications for the health status of local communities and for the health status of individuals within those communities. If these objectives are to be achieved, decentralization must be integral to decision-making and not be merely an after-the-event clip-on (tokenistic consultation once decisions have been made). And if this integration is to be complete, it must begin at the very start of the decision-making process. Decentralization must be built in from the process of policy formation through to the most detailed of operational considerations.

However, local health sector decision-making takes place within a broader context. This is a context in which other parties than the locality—generally those closer to the centre of national health systems—also have a legitimate interest. These may be contradictory to the local interest. These contradictions, if they are not to translate into outright conflict, must be tackled head-on and nowhere more importantly than within the various planning processes. It is the role of decentralised planning processes to ensure that all appropriate parties are represented and, even if they may not agree with the outcome of a particular decision, they should feel that the decision has been arrived at through legitimate process.

Designing such planning systems is no simple task. First, they must achieve an appropriate balance between the interests of the centre and the interest of the locality. Within the most advanced of health systems (particularly the British National Health Service), attempts to achieve more localised control have been thwarted by the concern that they will imperil the 'national' flavour of the health service. Second, they must ensure an appropriate balance between the urgency of the immediate and the importance of the longer term. This is most usually manifested in balancing the more curative needs of local health service delivery and the more preventive needs of maximising health gain through public health measures.

And planning systems must be 'joined-up'. A regular failing of health-care planning systems is that longer term plans (frequently formulated solely at the centre of the health-care system) are divorced from the shorter term planning process (which may or may not be devolved to the periphery). Thus, there is no mechanism to translate higher ideals (often formulated in the achievement, for example, of Millennium Development Goals) into operational decisions.

Planning Processes

Planning systems are generally portrayed as being cyclical in nature. Stages in the cycle (which we will consider in more detail below) are conventionally labelled 'situational analysis'; 'priority, goal and objective setting'; 'option appraisal'; 'programming'; 'implementation and monitoring'; and 'evaluation'. Some authors (Green 1992) prefer the term 'planning spiral' rather than 'planning cycle', emphasising the progressive nature of each turn in the cycle. They also stress the extent to which planning systems feed into and build upon each other.

Crudely, planning processes may be distinguished between the *strategic* and the *tactical*. The terms are by no means distinct, and the respective processes should certainly be blurred (or overlapping) in operation. Strategic planning involves integrating and operationalising long-term policy objectives with the outline process of resource allocation. Historically, strategic planning has tended to take place on a stand-alone 5- or 10-year planning horizon and is a process which has been undertaken exclusively at the centre of national health systems. Tactical planning takes place over a shorter planning horizons (generally a single year) and is executed at the regional and/or district level, depending upon the degree of decentralization. Traditionally, this involved deciding upon how the resources that have been 'handed down' from above will be allocated to the respective units (districts or facilities) within the planning bodies' jurisdiction. The term *operational planning* is also frequently encountered, though this tends to refer to periodic (say, three monthly) management decisions about relatively short-term utilisation of resources.

The separation of these processes generally leads to planning operating in staccato fashion giving rise to a sense of frustration. Each turn of the cycle is approached as an ab initio activity, discontinuous from its predecessor and from its successor. Prior to each new turn of the strategic planning cycle, an evaluation will be conducted, essentially a post-mortem on why the previous planning period's objectives have not been achieved. An alternate approach, providing for more continuity, is to view each separate planning period as part of a rolling horizon. Thus, at the strategic level, each 5-year period will lay down outline plans for the following 5-year period and indicative plans for the 5-year period following that. The process of evaluation will be executed periodically within the current planning period, so that outline and indicative plans are constantly reviewed in the light of current performance. Similarly, at the tactical level, annual plans will contain outline and indicative proposals for subsequent 1-year planning periods.

In addition to temporal integration (as above), functional integration requires the harmonisation of human resource, physical and financial planning processes. As it is the latter which generally constrains the first two, an element of iteration is required (as well as considerable overlap in the membership of planning bodies where these bodies are separate entities). Fuller consideration of these issues, which dictate the efficacy of all planning systems regardless of the degree of decentralization, can be found in a standard textbook of health planning (Green 1992).

Community Engagement in Planning

The degree of meaningful and effective community engagement is the ultimate measure of the impact of a decentralization programme. If, as we have implied above, decentralization is not seen as an end in its own right but as a means to more sensitive and thus more effective decision-making, community engagement becomes an integral part of the decentralization process—rather than a 'clip on' or a parallel process.

As the overall system is essentially hierarchical in nature—with policy formation setting the parameters for strategic planning which in turn sets the parameters for tactical and then operational planning—community involvement can frequently come at a very late stage. Communities may merely be asked to respond to proposals that have already been well considered and well argued and thus may (in the minds of more powerful decision-makers) be settled. Community involvement becomes tokenistic. The obstacles to engaging communities at a more formative stage are partly perceptual (reflecting dominant beliefs in professional roles) and partly reflective of the wider democratic structures within which the planning systems operate. Although forms of community involvement *may* be seen in more centralised political structures, which generally see communities as local providers of services, full community involvement in the health planning process is difficult to implement outside of a context of more generalised decentralised governance.

The precise form of community engagement, particularly the representative structures through which the community voice is accessed, will depend on the overall context of decentralization. Where powers across all sectors are fully decentralised and communities are meaningfully engaged, community involvement in health sector planning should operate through existing structures rather than require additional mechanisms. Thus the most effective forms of community engagement are those that operate through functioning systems of local governance.

Intersectoral Integration of Planning

A reservation frequently expressed against a full engagement of communities in the planning process is the concern that communities (or their representatives) will prioritise the urgent over the important, meaning that they will favour short-term measures aimed at improving the availability of curative health services over longer term measures designed to tackle the underlying determinants of poor health. Empirical evidence suggests that this fear is unfounded. For example, a community-led health planning exercise conducted within a deprived area of North Cork in the Republic of Ireland (NICHE 2003) identified eight 'themes for action' (a clean and beautiful environment; health and well-being; medical facilities and health services; children, young people and education; safe environment; housing; social, personal and community development; and recreational, sports and amenities), of which only one was service focused. Although, within these themes, the improvement of general practitioner services was accorded the highest priority (not unreasonably given their then paucity), this figured alongside very practical proposals for the improvement of the housing situation which had been allowed to run down over previous decades to the long-term detriment of the health of the community.

In practice, it is more usually the institutional response to communities' articulation of non-health service-focused priorities that inhibits communities from raising wider issues. Placing the health sector in a discrete organisational silo precludes professional health sector planners from providing an adequate response to non-health service issues. 'Yes, we recognise that environmental pollution is having a detrimental impact on the health of your community; but that is outside of our sphere of control'.

Implicitly, this exposes a very fundamental issue for the entire project of the decentralization of the health sector. This is whether, in practice, decentralization within a single sector is ever achievable without a full-scale programme of governmental decentralization. Notwithstanding that single-sector decentralization will pose cultural/perceptional dilemmas—'why should communities be allowed/expect/have faith in decentralised planning processes in one area whilst they remain centralised in others?'—decentralization within one sector will inevitably produce an imbalance in focus, concentrating on the mechanisms of health-care delivery rather than on the underlying determinants of poor health.

Integration across sectors has been considered a priority at global and national levels recently. Following from the formative work of the WHO's Commission on Social Determinants of Health (CSDH, 2008) and, more explicitly, from the Review of Health Inequalities within the UK led by Professor Sir Michael Marmot (2010), recognition of the need to plan health interventions across all sectors has been termed the *whole systems approach*. As well as acknowledging the importance of the inclusion of other sectors in planning for health improvement, the *whole systems approach* highlights the critical role of 'front-line' health service staff in achieving wider public health objectives. For example, the influence of midwives or traditional birth attendants in moulding the future health environment (rather than just the immediate outcome of the birthing process) renders their input critical to the formulation of longer term programmes addressing poor nutrition, poor housing conditions, positive health behaviours, etc. Decentralised planning systems must be inclusive within the health sector as well as being inclusive of other sectors and of local communities.

Case Study (Malawi)

In Malawi, a District Implementation Plan Process was introduced as part of the wider decentralization programme being introduced within the Ministry of Health and Population with support from the European Commission's Health Sector Reform and Decentralization Project. At the time, the health sector was seen as being a flagship ministry in the national decentralization

(continued)

(Continued)

programme which was designed to transfer powers, including the management of local health services, from central government to elected District Assemblies. Central to this was the formation and strengthening of District Health Management Teams.

The District Implementation Plan Process was an annual exercise. It was undertaken within broad parameters established within the then National Health Plan. The District Implementation Plan process began with districts revisiting their existing 5-year plans and revising them in accordance with national plan objectives. District planning guidelines (Republic of Malawi Ministry of Health and Population, 2000) were provided to districts, team members from which were instructed in their use at a series of workshops, and guided through a serious of structured exercises and worksheets. The output of this process, in addition to the district implementation plan itself, was an analysis of required resources and a monitoring and evaluation plan.

This planning process was innovative in a number of respects. First, it introduced districts to implementation as a rolling process. The implementation period for the first operation of the planning cycle was 1 July 2001 to 30 June 2002. But in drawing up these plans, districts were asked to ‘set the foundation’ for the periods 2002–2003 and 2003–2004. Rather than endeavouring to lump everything into the immediate year ahead, districts were explicitly required to prioritise. To assist in prioritisation (and in the clarification of the relationship between respective problems and objectives), districts were introduced to some specific techniques of problem structuring.

Following realignment of planned district activities with the objectives of the National Health Plan, district team members were asked to undertake a problem identification process in respect of local implementation—to *identify the problems that are keeping you from achieving the activities that you have listed under this objective*. On the basis of the problems identified, districts were asked to determine *actions* to overcome them. Districts then employed a mapping process designed to enable them to draw out the interconnections between individual actions and where possible to aggregate individual actions into *activity areas*.

The product of the mapping exercise was a re-aggregation of intended activities, providing district health management teams with a deeper understanding of the consequences (good and bad) of pursuing particular strategic courses of action. The mapping process clarified the problem space but still required districts to undertake a process of prioritisation and choice. To assist them with this, they were asked to undertake a ranking exercise.

A Decentralised Community-Focused Health Planning Spiral

It will be apparent from these general considerations that decentralised community-focused health planning is more challenging to implement than are the traditional 'top-down' approaches. It is not possible (nor appropriate) to offer a blueprint for decentralised health planning here. Rather we will consider the stages of the planning cycle (or planning spiral) as they are conventionally formulated and identify the special features that relate to a more decentralised system of planning. {Fuller articulation of these stages can be found in a standard text such as Green (1992)}. It is, however, worth restating a key feature that is stressed in planning texts. This is that, although the stages are generally presented sequentially, reflecting their general movement towards the formulation and implementation of firm planning decisions, the stages should be approached iteratively—revisiting an 'earlier' stage in the light of considerations that might transpire at subsequent stages. With the additional complexity of operating decentralised community-focused planning systems, such revisiting might be considered essential.

Situational Analysis

The situational analysis, as the name implies, involves a full assessment of the health status of local populations, variations within and between those populations, the determinants of that health situation and the nature of and context within which health care is currently being delivered. A decentralised community-focused health planning system will adopt a more expansive and possibly (though not necessarily) more exhaustive approach to the associated data collection.

Most critically, such a system will require data that are not obtainable from within formal data systems. Although formal systems may provide the necessary patterns of epidemiology, demography, resource availability and distribution and (to some extent) pertinent environmental features, they can only hint at the translation of these into patterns of community perception, community prioritisation and community utilisation. To investigate these issues further, some authors have advocated the adoption of *rapid appraisal* approaches (Annett and Rifkin 1995). For access to 'hard-to-reach' communities, a system of *key informants* may be established. These approaches will be considered further in the accompanying chapter on measurement.

In the operation of a rolling health planning system, the process of data collection becomes progressively more straightforward. Rather than collecting all information ab initio at every turn of the spiral, data collection focuses on updating key indicators—a feature that we will return to later in this chapter and which is also considered more fully in the accompanying chapter.

Priority, Goal and Objective Setting

The priority-setting stage encompasses deciding upon what we want from our health sector and the relative importance of respective calls on resources. Terminologies vary, though this essentially constitutes establishing a *hierarchy of objectives*—an ordering between long-, medium- and short-term objectives with specification of their interconnectedness. Although it may be relatively easy to agree higher order objectives (or, in the case say of the local implementation of Millennium Development Goals, these may be translated down), it is the priority accorded to respective determining factors that will be more contentious and will call for widest involvement.

First, there will be variation in perspectives on the relative urgency or importance of measures as we have highlighted above. These may be driven by or accentuated by legitimate (and sometimes not-so-legitimate) sectional interests. As well as the obvious differences that may be accorded by different demographic sections of the community (which don't necessarily play out as might be predicted) or by different geographically situated sections of the community (urban/rural, say), there will be differing priorities accorded to the needs of more marginal sections of the community. Centralised planning systems have a tendency to sweep such issues under the carpet—often fuelling resentment and inter-communal conflict in the process. Decentralised community-focused planning systems must incorporate processes by which they may be explicitly drawn out—in practice frequently revealing more generosity of spirit than may have been pre-assumed.

Option Appraisal

The adoption of a *whole systems approach* incorporates a much richer view of the causation of poor and good health status. It also heightens considerably the complexity of selecting options between the competing routes for attaining agreed objectives—the purpose of the option appraisal stage. This was demonstrated most forcefully by the work of the Foresight Committee which undertook a review of the strategies for tackling obesity within the UK (Butland et al. 2007). Central to their recommendations was an *obesity map* showing the various influences impacting upon what has been conceived as the current obesity epidemic. In its initial formulation (called the *full generic obesity map*) this was so detailed and so complex that it was illegible to the naked eye. However, subsequent work by the team (undertaking what might be called systems analysis, see below) rendered this complexity more manageable and more meaningful and provided a substantive basis through which the varying paths and routes might be addressed.

Option appraisal involves not only the identification but also the evaluation of the different available paths for reaching desired objectives. This includes both economic and non-economic dimensions (Green 1992). When planning is undertaken in a traditional top-down non-participatory way, the economic dimension will appear as a constraint imposed upon the aspirations of the locality from above. In a more participative mode, the economic appraisal will be seen as a mutual recognition of the need to allocate (necessarily) scarce resource most effectively. However, the major benefit of decentralised community-focused planning is that it enables the non-economic dimensions to be accorded appropriate emphasis. Thus, local cultural considerations or local behavioural constraints can be taken into account from the start rather than appearing as obstacles to be circumvented as remotely developed and locally insensitive plans are implemented.

Programming

The adoption of a rolling approach, as advocated above, can ease the process of programming. Rather than options being simply ruled 'in' or 'out', those which are accorded lesser importance or urgency can be programmed to outline or indicative status, signalling provisional allocation to subsequent planning periods. The danger of putting the important issues on hold pending completion of those which are deemed urgent remains, but it does avoid them being taken off of the agenda entirely, and it does draw out explicitly the inherent tension between the two.

Programming activities in a participative fashion permits a realistic identification of the respective contribution of different agencies. This will hopefully avoid the frustrations that can result from the unrealistic expectations of the contribution from other sectors (or from the community itself) that can result from centrally generated plans.

Implementation and Monitoring

This will necessarily ease the transition from programming to implementation as these agencies will already be signed up to proposals.

A decentralised community-focused planning system will reflect greater balance at the monitoring stage in keeping with the richer situational analysis outlined above. This will result in closer tracking of both quantitative and qualitative dimensions of programme implementation. Again, *key informants* can be employed to provide information on otherwise hard-to-reach parts of the broad health-care system.

Evaluation

The evaluation stage is critical within any planning system but it is all-too-frequently viewed as an external after-the-event activity rather than as an organic part of the planning process. Whereas external involvement can be extremely valuable at the evaluation stage—in providing a greater degree of objectivity and in marrying the lessons of a particular implementation with those from elsewhere—it should be driven by the full range of data being generated by programme monitoring, as well as specially commissioned data collection which might address the broader impact. Below, we will consider use of the logical framework which if carefully formulated can ensure that all appropriate considerations are drawn out in the evaluation stage.

Scenario: Case Study (Malawi)

As a member of the District Health Management Team for the Nzonga District of Malawi, you are engaged in the District Implementation Plan Process.

Your district is located in the northern region of Malawi. It is some distance from Lilongwe and Blantyre, the two major urban centres. As a consequence, recruitment and retention of all cadres of staff is a persistent problem for the district.

The district has recently experienced high levels of maternal and infant mortality and morbidity. Analysis of the root causes has prompted the pursuit of a two-pronged strategy:

1. Improvement of maternal health through improved access to quality health services
2. Improvement in the quality and access to family planning services

A number of issues have been identified impeding progress in each of the respective areas:

1. Improving education in the causes of poor maternal and child health is known to be crucial for reducing maternal and child morbidity and mortality, but the ability to implement this is constrained by the availability of appropriate educational materials, insufficient transport to access outlying areas within the district and the availability of a generator to power a video and PA system in areas without mains electricity. Within health facilities, there is a shortage of trained staff sufficiently skilled to undertake educational and preventive activities, and the availability of basic delivery and sterilisation equipment is limited. Most deliveries in the district are currently performed by birth assistants, few of whom are trained in appropriate safe motherhood and few of whom receive any supervision from members of the district health management team. The ability to supervise is constrained by shortage of transport or available transport being in a state of disrepair. Better telephone and radio communication might replace direct supervision, but the appropriate equipment is not currently available in the district. Better telecommunication equipment would also help to

(continued)

notify health facilities when there is an obstetric emergency in the community, though shortage of transport would constrain the ability to respond within an appropriate timescale. Given the limited contact between members of the district health management team and the birth attendants undertaking deliveries, information on the birthing process is limited. When a maternal or child death occurs, there is currently no follow-up.

2. The reasons why the demand for family planning in the district is currently very low are not well known, but it is known that there are problems in the supply chain as a consequence of the shortage of static or mobile local family planning facilities. It is felt that not sufficient use is made of current health service contacts with both women and men to inform them on the benefits of contraception. There are few health facilities that currently provide a base for family planning, and community-based staff and members of village health committees are generally not knowledgeable of the benefits of contraception. Community-based information programmes have historically been obstructed by religious leaders who see them as a threat to local practices which are generally conservative in nature; current health workers are insufficiently trained to counter their arguments. Information on the provision and utilisation of contraception is generally poor, with weak communication between the district health management team and community-based maternity services and only occasional supervision. When men and women do begin to practice contraception, there is little follow-up and a lack of information on whether practices are sustained.

Tools to Assist Decentralised Planning

Planning Toolkits

This chapter does not offer a manual for a decentralised community-focused planning system. Frequent reference has been made to appropriate textbooks (particularly Green 1992) which allow for fuller consideration of planning processes more generally. Attempts to formulate manuals for a decentralised planning process, or for components of it, have been made. {These should not be confused with, for example, Management Science for Health's *Decentralization Planning Tool* (Kolehmainen-Aitken 1999) which is designed to aid the process of planning decentralization rather than processes of planning within a decentralised context.}

Save the Children's *Toolkits* (Gosling and Edwards 1995) provides a compendium of methods that can be employed within the planning cycle when approached in a participatory style. Particular focus has been applied to the use of rapid methods for data collection and health needs assessment. Kielmann et al (1992) offer a comprehensive set of assessment protocols; Annett and Rifkin (1995) present guidelines for the process of conducting a community health needs assessment.

Problem Structuring Approaches to Decentralised Health Planning

Problem structuring methods have evolved as a distinct body of operational research modelling techniques as a response to the discipline's traditional focus on quantitative approaches. These were perceived to treat 'messy' unstructured problem contexts, such as decentralised health-care systems, as if they were well structured. This resulted in inappropriate or simplistic representations which involved selectively fitting problem characteristics to available analytic techniques generally at the expense of more important features of the problem context. Operational research practitioners borrowed from elsewhere, particularly from the worlds of planning and systems theory, to produce a new range of modelling techniques (sometimes referred to as 'soft OR'). These depended on much less quantitative data and used a wider range of conceptual (qualitative) modelling approaches. Classic examples are the Strategic Choice Approach, with its roots in partnership planning, and Strategic Options Development and Analysis, with its roots in personal construct theory and cognitive mapping. {A discussion of the origins of problem structuring methods and an introduction to some of the most frequently employed techniques can be found in Rosenhead and Mingers (2001); though, see also Flood and Jackson (1991), Bryant (1989) and Taket and White (2000)}. The essence of the problem structuring approach is not to shoehorn problems into an available analytic technique (which had been seen as a frequent failing of conventional operational research) but to borrow widely and to adapt freely, as the situation requires.

Mapping

The complexities of the competing means through which the agreed objectives of a local community might be achieved provide as complex a problem context as that revealed by the Foresight Committee as bearing on the national issue of obesity in the UK. Visual representations of these complexities can be beneficial in understanding the alternate approaches that might be adopted, notwithstanding how confusing they might initially appear. Thunhurst (2007) considers the use of mapping techniques to assist the analysis of visual maps. Drawing upon work undertaken in the Republic of Ireland, a planning context exhibiting some areas of potentially acute conflict was restructured to distinguish substantive disagreements from the superficial and to highlight areas of agreement that were initially overshadowed by the areas of disagreement.

Thunhurst and Barker (1999) outline approaches that were initially developed in Pakistan and subsequently incorporated into the decentralised health planning system in Malawi (see Box 6.1). Mapping was employed within the Malawian District Implementation Plan Process and described in the following terms:

> 'Mapping establishes relationships between potential health service actions. It helps to clarify which actions need to be considered in conjunction, and whether it is critical that one action must necessarily precede another. Where groups of actions are interdependent, this

Box 6.1 Planning Exercise 1: Case Study (Malawi)

Consider the scenario presented in the Malawi Case Study above. Identify objectives which might be included within your district implementation plan for the coming year and show the relationship between them, where they are interrelated. Be sure to take account of the necessary implementation period (short, medium or long term) and any sequential relationships between objectives.

group may be defined as an **activity area**. Mapping will thus provide a shortened list of activity areas. It will indicate that some activities cannot be considered before other activities have been carried out to create appropriate conditions. Other activities will perhaps emerge as priorities. A note may be made of this, but any indications about time sequence should be considered in relation to the results, which are gained, in the total process. A line is drawn on the map, when there is a significant possibility of a different outcome if two activities are considered together. If the group judges that two activities must be considered together and that one must occur before the other, a directional arrow may be drawn.' Republic of Malawi Ministry of Health and Population (2000)

Figure 6.1, below, demonstrates how one district used such an approach to analyse the interrelationships between factors affecting the performance of their family planning programme.

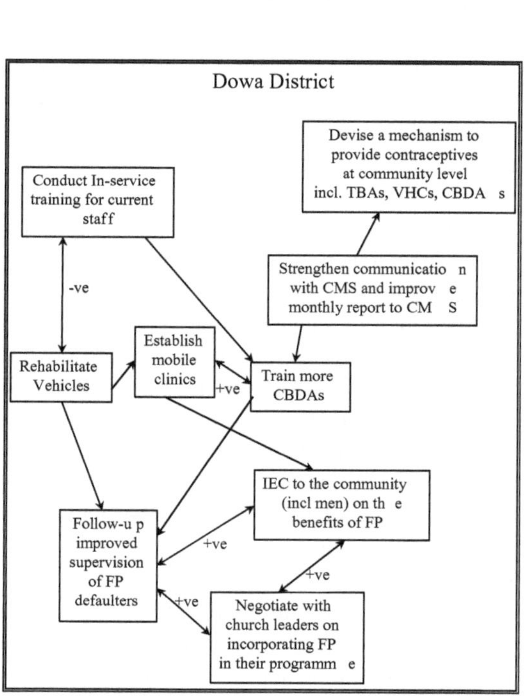

Fig. 6.1 A district-level activity map

Ranking

Mapping was thereby employed as a first step in option appraisal allowing fuller elaboration of the consequences (intended and unintended) of competing option paths. This will not necessarily (indeed, will rarely) make selection between options easier. To assist this stage in the process the Malawian District Implementation Plan Process incorporated a mechanism for ranking options. This was described in the following terms.

> 'Activity areas and potential health service actions can be further structured using a ranking method. There are many examples of ranking systems in health care planning. Ranking allows quite different types of consideration to be integrated into a priority-setting process. The approach involves the group doing the ranking first, reviewing what criteria are important to them, and agreeing an evaluation procedure. The process of discussing criteria and making a group judgement about what is most important is an essential feature of this process. Any weightings need to be agreed in advance for each criterion. Weightings are highly dependent upon local circumstances e.g. budgetary availability, socio-political context; and should not be generalized.' Republic of Malawi Ministry of Health and Population (2000)

Table 6.1 shows the exemplar pro forma that was included in the planning guidelines (Republic of Malawi Ministry of Health and Population, 2000) to assist district teams to establish their own priorities.

The Logical Framework Approach

A view that we have frequently heard expressed when being introduced to the planning systems operating within specific developing countries is that 'we are very good at planning, but we are not very good at implementation'. Resisting the temptation to respond 'in that case, you're not very good at planning', the observation was taken as recognition of the difficulties encountered in moving from intention to delivery. Frequently the obstacles are political in nature, with paper agreement being easier to achieve than commitment to change in practice. These can be reduced (though not fully eliminated) by ensuring the participative nature of the planning process, thereby ensuring that all parties are, nominally at least, 'signed up'. But equally frequently the obstacles do represent a failure within the planning system of separating the decision-making stages of the planning process from the implementation and monitoring stages.

A well-tried mechanism for strengthening this process of translation is the *Logical Framework*. In operational research/systems analysis terms, the logical framework can be thought of as a *model* of the plan—a simplified representation which captures, in a structured format, critical outcomes of the planning process. But it also provides a checklist, ensuring that planning outcomes are fully thought through and are capable of being implemented and monitored. Although initially conceived as a project planning and implementation tool, it has been widely adopted and adapted for use within the wider tactical and strategic planning contexts (Table 6.2).

Table 6.1 Ranking pro forma used to aid prioritisation

	Possible interventions		
Ranking criteria	Career development/ training	Incentives to work in rural areas	Improve supervision
How important is the issue?			
Is change in this area feasible?	++	+	++
How urgent is the issue?	++	++	+++
How large is the population group affected by this policy?	+++	+++	+++
How much of health activity is affected by this policy?	++	++	++
How popular would resulting improvements be?	+	+++	+++
B. What is the cost of change and the cost of no change?			
Will change cost money?	--	---	--
Will change save money?	+	+	++
Will change cost staff time?	--	-	--
Will change save staff time?	++	+	++
Will change cost effort in management and planning	--	--	--
Will change save effort in management and planning?	+	+	++
C. Does this policy area affect:			
Accessibility	++	++	+++
Long-term credibility	+++	++	+++
Efficiency	+++	++	+++
Equity	+	++	+
Quality of services	++	++	+++
D. Does this strategic option require involvement of other sectors?		**	

Put most simply, the logical framework is a four-by-four matrix. Although, the precise titling of the columns may vary, the first column (often called the *narrative summary*) records the hierarchy of objectives—goal, purpose, outputs and activities—of the project/plan. The *goal* is an expression of the wider intention of the project/plan, generally tying it into higher order planning processes (Millennium Development Goals, national planning objectives). The *purpose* is a statement of the intended impact of a project/plan—what will change in the broader environment as a consequence of the project/plan's successful implementation. This may be distinguished from the *outputs* which may be thought of as the project/plan's deliverables which, for all but the most simple projects, will be several (but ideally less than six). The *outputs* will reflect specific changes that will have been achieved by the end of the project/plan period. *Activities*, which are specifically linked to each individual output, provide a breakdown of these into operational detail (enabling fuller articulation of areas of responsibility).

Table 6.2 The logical framework

Narrative summary (NS)	Verifiable indicators (OVI)	Means of verification (MoV)	Important assumptions
Goal			
Purpose			
Outputs			
1.			
2.			
3.			
4.			
5.			
Activities			
1.1			
1.2			
:			
:			
2.1			
2.2			
:			
:			
3.1			
3.2			
:			
:			
:			
:			

The second column of the logical framework lists (observable) verifiable indicators. At each level of the hierarchy of objectives and against individual outputs and activities, a number of specific indicators will be listed enabling an objective assessment of whether the objective has been achieved. There is a traditional preference for quantitative indicators, given the greater ease of measurement and comparison that these provide. But an undue concentration on quantitative indicators may fail to capture the richness of project/plan intention, particularly where process change is being sought.

The third column of the logical framework specifies means of verification. This provides for a check against individual indicators that a source of data enabling calibration of the indicator either exists or can be established without initiating a disproportionate data collection exercise.

The final column records any Important Assumptions built into the project/plan. Except in trivial implementations, progress through the hierarchy of objectives (converting activities into outputs, converting outputs into purpose, etc.) will be dependent upon the cooperation of other agencies or upon either change or stability in the external environment. Such issues are essentially out of project/plan control. Assumptions can be tested to ensure that they are not unrealistic or to see whether project/plan design should be modified to ensure that they are explicitly addressed within the project/plan.

In a context within which planning has been undertaken previously in a top-down hierarchical fashion, the logical framework may expose the inadequacy of existing information systems. Decentralised community-focused health planning requires monitoring change at the community level which may not be built into current information systems. We will return to the nature of community-focused health indictors in a subsequent chapter, but it is likely that the construction of new systems will stand outside the remit of an individual planning body or the timescale of an individual planning period.

Planning Exercise 2: Case Study (Malawi)

Drawing upon the objectives identified in Planning Exercise 1 above, establish a hierarchy of objectives. Identify priorities for the coming year and objectives that you would signpost for inclusion in medium- (5-year) and long-term (10-year) outline plans. Identify the relationship between the objectives for the coming year and those being pursued in the medium and longer term.

Discussion and Summary

The greatest challenge to integrated community-focused health planning in developing countries is the continued existence of separate nationally directed vertical programmes. Their retention often reflects the lack of confidence from external donors in local mechanisms of implementation and monitoring. However, insistence on the maintenance of separate parallel systems can only ultimately serve to weaken these mechanisms, creating a self-fulfilling prophecy and thereby undermining the broader decentralization programme that the same donors may generally profess to support. More legitimately, vertical programmes are frequently viewed as areas of excellence which must be protected. In practice, it is more often the empires surrounding the programmes which are being protected, as vertical programmes are generally more generously funded than is 'routine' health-care delivery.

A commitment to move to the integration of separate vertical programmes is the strongest statement of intent in respect of decentralization that national health sector policy formers can make. It is also therefore the best indicator available of the degree of political support to the wider decentralization programme. Throughout this chapter, it has been stressed that decentralization of health planning can only be effectively realised where there is a strong commitment to genuine community involvement and where there exist operational decentralised intersectoral planning mechanisms. These two conditions necessitate drawing into the health planning process agencies and individuals who have no previous experience of health sector planning. If they are given the appropriate freedoms, this will be a refreshing experience for health sector planners enabling them to break out of their historical focus on health services planning. However, it will also require an intensive induction process.

Some of the techniques presented above will be unfamiliar to existing professional health planners, let alone to planners from other sectors and to representatives of communities that are drawn into the planning process. The techniques themselves are not intrinsically complex but, at the initial stages at least, will require some facilitation. This in turn becomes the primary role for health planners within the health sector—facilitating the wider engagement that community-focused decentralised health planning requires. The introduction of decentralised health planning must be accompanied by a human resource development plan for health sector planners. And it is in respect of this function that intermediary (regional) levels will have their most important role, providing institutional support to the decentralization process at the locality level.

Recommended Reading

Green, A. (1992). *An introduction to health planning in developing countries*. Oxford: Oxford University Press.

A comprehensive and structured introduction to methods of and issues relating to health planning in developing countries, introducing the planning cycle and taking the reader through the respective stages of the cycle.

Marmot, M. (2010). Fair society, Healthy lives. *The Marmot Review*. London: The Marmot Review. Available through: www.ucl.ac.uk/marmotreview

Chapter 5 of The Marmot Review, entitled Making it happen *provides an explanation of the meaning and the importance of adopting a Whole Systems Approach with examples of how such an approach might be operationalised.*

Butland, B., Jebb, S., Kopelman, P., McPherson, K., Thomas, S., Mardell, J., & Parry, V. (2007). *Foresight—Tackling obesities: Future choices*. London: Government Office for Science. Available at: http://www.bis.gov.uk/assets/foresight/docs/obesity/17.pdf

The Foresight Report on tackling obesity provides comprehensive illustration of how a complex problem context can be analysed using mapping and systems analysis.

Rosenhead, J., & Mingers, J. (2001). Rational analysis for a problematic world revisited. Chichester: Wiley.

Provides both a general introduction and some specific examples of the new paradigm Problem Structuring Methods of Operational Research/Systems Analysis. Description of each technique is accompanied by a practical example of its use.

References

Annett, H., & Rifkin, S. (1995). *Guidelines for rapid appraisals to assess community health needs WHO/SHS/DHS/958*. Geneva: WHO.

Bryant, J. (1989). *Problem management—a guide for producers and players*. Chichester: Wiley.

Butland, B., Jebb, S., Kopelman, P., McPherson, K., Thomas, S., Mardell, J., & Parry, V. (2007). *Foresight—tackling obesities: Future choices*. London: Government Office for Science.

CSDH. (2008). *Closing the gap in a generation: Health equity through action on the social determinants of health. Final Report of the Commission on Social Determinants of Health*. Geneva: World Health Organization. Available through: http://www.who.int/social_determinants/the-commission/en/index.html.

Flood, R., & Jackson, M. (1991). *Creative problem solving—Total systems intervention*. Chichester: Wiley.

Gosling, L., & Edwards, M. (1995). *Toolkits—A practical guide to assessment, monitoring, review and evaluation*. London: Save the Children.

Green, A. (1992). *An introduction to health planning in developing countries*. Oxford: Oxford University Press.

Kielmann, A., Janovsky, K., & Annett, H. (1992). *Assessing district health needs, services and systems—Protocols for rapid data collection and analysis*. London: AMREF and Macmillan.

Kolehmainen-Aitken, R.-L. (1999). *The decentralization planning tool*. Boston: Management Sciences for Health.

Marmot, M. (2010). *Fair society, healthy lives. The Marmot Review*. London: The Marmot Review.

NICHE. (2003). *Knocknaheeny/Hollyhill Community Health Planning Report 2003*. Cork, RoI: Northside Initiative for Community Health.

Rosenhead, J., & Mingers, J. (2001). *Rational analysis for a problematic world revisited*. Chichester: Wiley.

Republic of Malawi Ministry of Health and Population. (2000). *District planning guidelines*. Lilongwe: MoHP.

Taket, A., & White, L. (2000). *Partnership and participation—Decision-making in the multiagency setting*. Chichester: Wiley.

Thunhurst, C. (2007). Refocusing upstream—Operational research for population health. *Journal of the Operational Research Society, 58*(186–194), 2007.

Thunhurst, C., & Barker, C. (1999). Using problem structuring methods in strategic planning. *Health Policy & Planning, 14*(2), 127–134.

Chapter 7
Measuring Health and Health Services

Colin Thunhurst

Abstract This chapter will help you to determine the nature and the size of the data set that is required to assess the efficient and efficacious working of a decentralised health system. It will introduce some general principles in the development of health information systems and consider their particular relevance to the monitoring and evaluation of decentralised systems. It will assist you in the selection of key indicators employing (for illustration) the logical framework as a key instrument. It will help you to assess the appropriateness of methods of data analysis and reporting and to determine appropriate methods and channels of feedback to decision-makers and data providers.

After Reading This Chapter You Will Be Able to

- *Understand the importance of building appropriate measurement into decentralised management and planning systems.*
- *Identify indicators appropriate to the monitoring and evaluation of a decentralised health-care system.*
- *Select appropriate methods of data analysis and presentation.*
- *Identify appropriate mechanisms and processes of information feedback.*

C. Thunhurst (✉)
Faculty of Health and Life Sciences, University of Coventry,
Stone Cottage, 5 Aire View, Sandbeds, Keighley, West Yorkshire, BD20 5LH, UK
e-mail: c.thunhurst@coventry.ac.uk

K. Regmi (ed.), *Decentralizing Health Services: A Global Perspective*,
DOI 10.1007/978-1-4614-9071-5_7,

Introduction

Too Much Data: Too Little Information

A regular feature and regular fault of Health Information Systems and Health Management Information Systems is that they are developed on a consensual basis which starts with a completely blank sheet. Posed with the abstract question 'what data should we collect', the inevitable response is 'everything'. The reasons for including items of data are always much stronger than the reasons for excluding them—in the absence of any clear criteria of choice. The inevitable consequence is *data overload*—the collection and storage of large quantities of data which are never analysed, or if analysed never used to inform any decision-making process. In the modern world of seemingly limitless data storage and analysis capacity, this may initially appear to pose no problem—does it matter that data are collected and end up just sitting in neglected data files (as it frequently in pre-computer days ended up sitting on dusty shelves)? But, if allowed to continue, systemic data underutilisation will jeopardise the quality of the really important material hidden within data sets—the data that *could be* analysed and used to inform the decision-making process. If data providers see as a regular occurrence that data that they are taking time and trouble to collect and to report are not being used for any meaningful purpose, they will (understandably) come to the conclusion that taking time and trouble isn't worth the effort—with the consequence that they will just submit any old numbers, because 'nobody bothers to use them', or they won't bother to submit data at all. All too frequently (in both developed and developing health systems) one encounters the vicious spiral of data degradation. Data analysts say 'we can't use the data that are provided to inform decision-making because they are unreliable and incomplete' and data providers say 'there's no use in providing accurate timely data because nobody ever uses them'. No data should be collected unless there is a clear and widely known use to which those data are to be put.

Decision-Making-Driven Information Systems

All information systems should be designed on the basis of a clear understanding of the decision-making processes that the data are being collected and analysed to support. For this, it is useful to start with some clear distinctions and differentiations.

Data, Information, Evidence and Decisions

Data are the raw numbers or words that appear in a data file, often in the form of a spreadsheet, though qualitative data may be stored in more narrative form (letters, supervisory reports, etc.). Data, on their own, have little value. Data attain value when they are analysed, enabling information to be extracted. A simple histogram may turn a set of data into information about the pattern (or distribution) of the prevalence of a disease, or its determinants, or of the way that resources are being used to counter it. But this information will be of little use (or of only academic use) if it is not fed into the decision-making process—providing what is now generally termed *evidence*. This is where the design of information systems should start, with a clear understanding of the decisions that will result from the process of data collection and analysis and from information dissemination. It may not be possible to get this right from the outset. Information needs may emerge as the decision-making process becomes more evidence driven, and this may necessitate revisiting the data collection and analysis that is undertaken. Information systems must have a degree of flexibility—incorporating periodic revision. But they should *not* be subject to constant tinkering—as too much change will jeopardise historic continuity, itself a valuable feature of an evidence base.

Health Information Systems and Health Management Information Systems

Although in practice there may be no clear distinction between the two, in terms of data collection, analysis and reporting systems, it is helpful to distinguish between two elements of the decentralised information system.

A *Health Information System* will consist of epidemiological data and associated analytic processes. It will be critical to the *situational analysis* stage of the planning cycle (p. 98, Chap. 6, above). It will have a more exploratory purpose in that it should alert decision-makers to emerging health issues and enable investigation of associated and determining factors. It is therefore important that it can easily be linked to parallel data sources containing information on salient features of the social, economic and environmental context. (A frequent problem experienced within developed countries such as the UK is that health is organised according to different administrative boundaries than local governance—General Practice Boundaries or Primary Care Trust boundaries. This can create major problems for data alignment and introduce issues of fuzziness into data analysis processes.) Key social, economic and environmental variables may be included within the health information system where they can give a succinct summary of the nature of the populations being served.

In contrast to the Health Information System, the *Health Management Information System* will be primarily concerned with resource utilisation. Its purpose is to enable decision-makers to identify where resources are being efficiently and inefficiently deployed and enable redeployment accordingly. It will be of particular relevance at the *programming* and *implementation and monitoring* stages of the planning cycle (p. 100, Chap. 6, above), and if given appropriate prior thought provide the necessary information for the *evaluation* stage. Health sector resources are generally classified as being financial, physical or human in nature; all of these should be adequately covered. Within a decentralised context, where community engagement is being explicitly fostered, it should also be comprehensive in that it should permit identification of appropriate resources in the community (such as voluntary health groups) and by corollary permit identification of where community-based resources are lacking and might require encouragement and/or development.

Data Quality

We have already considered the importance of ensuring data quality so as to avoid the vicious cycle whereby data which are not utilised can rapidly turn into data which are not usable. Central to ensuring that data remain to be of high quality is provision of regular feedback to data providers. We will consider appropriate mechanism of information feedback below, but the general rule should be that all reported data should be acted upon regardless of the immediate reliability that can be placed upon them (if subsequent data revision is necessary, so be it; this can in many respects be a good sign to data providers of the importance that is accorded to the data that they are providing).

On a visit to Tanzania I was discussing the value of good health information systems with a regional health officer. Dismissively, he told me that he had recently received a report from one district saying that there had been 12 cases of smallpox in the preceding month. "What did you do with the report?" I asked him. "Well, of course I threw it away—the data were clearly fictitious" he replied. "Why did you do that?", I asked him; "If you had gone back to the district and asked them what they were doing about the 12 cases of smallpox in their district they would have taken more care about their data reporting in the future".

Linking Measurement to Planning and Management Systems

Core Indicators

The critical link between data collection and analysis and the use of information to provide evidence to support decision-making is the identification of appropriate *indicators*. Sometimes the choice of an appropriate indicator will be relatively straightforward. For monitoring the performance of a disease-focussed programme, it will be necessary to have a clear knowledge of prevalence rates and of their distribution. But selecting indicators to monitor the effectiveness of more complex systemic interventions, of the sort that come from adopting a *whole systems* view, (as introduced in Chap. 6, above), will be more difficult. A whole systems perspective might lead us to feel, for example, that the subsidisation of public transport might have far-reaching positive health impacts. However, these impacts are likely to be spread across a number of specific health conditions—most directly, for example, a reduction in the number of childhood road traffic accidents; or a decrease in heart diseases (as the streets become more walker and cyclist friendly); or a reduction in rates of depression due to the isolation of the elderly. It is also possible that positive health impacts will only be achieved if the measure is accompanied by accompanying actions from other implementing agencies. If the easier traffic flows that come from shifting people from private to public transport lead to an increase in traffic speed, this could have the opposite impact on childhood accidents than was intended. (These are generally referred to as perverse consequences.) So, out of this web of potential interacting interventions, parallel policies and their respective diverse outcomes, how do we extract one (or a small set) of indicators to enable us to monitor and evaluate specific proposals in a way that won't lead to their impact being swamped and thereby hidden by confounding background noise?

Necessarily, the answer will involve an element of judgement and an element of compromise. Decisions on appropriate indicators within such a complex context are best arrived at following a process of inclusive discussion. This can be most productive if it is initiated by considering the pertinent causal processes—what might be the good (and bad) health impacts of a proposed measure? How might these impacts be maximised (or mitigated)? What might get in the way of achieving desired impacts and what parallel measures might be needed to avert them? Such consideration can lead to the production of a *causal map* (p. 104, Chap. 6, above) from which we can identify critical decision points, intermediary influences and likely end points. At each of these, we would want to define an appropriate indicator, thereby producing what would be known as a *core set of indicators*.

A good example of the process of developing a core set of indicators is given in Parkinson (2012). A good example of a full set of core indicators is given in Rigby and Köhler (2002) (Table 7.1).

We may also need to recognise that our first iteration at indicator definition might be constrained by data availability. The complexity of the social, economic and environmental context (what we will call the *upstream*) is such that we will frequently need to rely upon data available from other sources, as collecting our own data would be financially and/or practically prohibitive—data on social isolation amongst the elderly, for example. Indicators do precisely what their name suggests—they indicate. Sometimes it will be necessary to use data from an available related source—what we would call a *surrogate indicator*—measuring something which is closely related to our immediate object of interest. It is unlikely that social isolation amongst the elderly will be directly measured, but rates of depression probably will be. Such fuzziness in our information set should be acknowledged and interpreted with appropriate caution in any conclusions that we might draw.

Objectives and their associated indicators may be quantitative or qualitative in nature, but they share the common feature that it must be possible to assess them and their achievement. Qualitative aspects may be directly assessable through the use of devices such as checklists or rating scales. Or they may be assessed indirectly through the use of surrogate single or composite indicators. In the context of a decentralised bottom-up planning system, community perceptions will form an essential component of 'success' or 'failure' and can be systematically analysed.

Table 7.1 The child health indicators of life and development (CHILD) indicator set

A. Demographic and socio-economic	B. Child health status, well-being	C. Health determinants, risk and protective factors	D. Child health systems and policy
1. Socio-economic circumstances 2. Children in poverty 3. Parental educational attainment 4. Child in single-parent households 5. Asylum seekers	**Child mortality** 1. Child mortality rates 2. Selected cause-specific mortality **Child morbidity** 3. Cancer 4. Diabetes 5. Asthma 6. Infectious diseases 7. Dental morbidity **Injuries to children** 8. Burns necessitating admission 9. Poisoning necessitating admission 10. Fracture of long bones **Mental health of children** 11. Attempted suicide	**Parental determinants** 1. Breastfeeding 2. Household environmental tobacco 3. Parental support **Child lifestyle determinants** 4. Physical activity 5. Tobacco smoking 6. Alcohol abuse 7. Substance misuse **Other factors** 8. Overweight and obesity 9. Children in care 10. Early school leavers 11. Educational enrolment 12. Air pollution exposure	1. Marginalised children's health care 2. Parental inpatient accompaniment **Health system quality** 3. Immunisation coverage 4. Leukaemia 5-year survival **Social policy indicators** 5. Physical punishment 6. Anti-bullying policies in schools **Physical protection policy** 7. Child transportation safety 8. Exposure to lead 9. Exposure to hazardous noise 10. Environmental tobacco smoke

Source: Rigby and Köhler (2002)

The Logical Framework as a Vehicle for Defining Core Indicators

It will be evident from the preceding discussion that defining a core set of indicators for the monitoring of an upstream intervention can be a complicated process. There will always be difficult decisions to make, but these can be structured and made more inclusive if these decisions are drawn out explicitly. A good vehicle for this is the logical framework that we introduced previously (pp. 105–108, Chap. 6, above).

The hierarchy of objectives recorded in the narrative summary can be used to capture the desired causal chain (extracted from the causal map). A set of proposed interventions (the activities) is aimed to have a number of direct consequences (the outputs), all of which are aimed at securing a desired impact (the purpose) leading to an ultimate health improvement (the goal).

The final (fourth) column of the framework is used to show where progression up through the hierarchy of objectives is dependent upon the policies or actions of other agencies—thus, in the example we have given above, achievement of higher order objectives might be dependent upon a local council introducing better traffic calming measures. This should be clearly stated and the likelihood of its occurrence assessed. If the assumption is very critical and if the likelihood is not strong, some adjustment to the intervention might be needed—either to increase the likelihood or to reduce the criticality of the assumption.

However, it is the second and third columns of the framework that are of particular relevance to our current consideration of issues of measurement. In the second column, against each individual objective listed in the first column, will be specified one or more *indicators* which will enable us to assess whether that objective has been met. For lower order objectives (activities or outputs), the indicators will be relatively instrumental. For higher order objectives, it may be necessary to adopt composite indicators reflecting the multidimensional nature of the concepts, such as health, that might lie at the core of the objectives.

For all indicators, but especially for those measuring the attainment of higher order objectives, it is important to ensure that appropriate sources of data to calibrate the indicators are available or that the data can be collected at practicable cost. The third column (the means of verification) of the framework will specify the source of data against each individual indicator listed in column two.

The elegance of this form of representation is that the lower half of the second and third columns—the indicators and their means of verification specified against activity and output level objectives—provides the monitoring system for the proposed intervention. The upper half—the indicators and their means of verification specified against purpose and goal level objectives—provides the evaluation system for the proposed intervention (Tables 7.2 and 7.3).

Core Indicators as a Vehicle for Clarifying Objectives

It can be seen that, by following the process identified above, the issues of measurement become integral to the design, monitoring and evaluation of proposed interventions. Measurement is embedded into the planning process. This can have concomitant beneficial effects. By asking the questions 'How do you intend to measure the achievement of this objective?' and 'What source of data do you intend to use?', the intended logic and progression that lie behind complex interventions can be sharpened.

Measurement should not be viewed as an 'after the event' consideration within the planning process—at either the design or implementation stages. It is a frequent misconception that the process of evaluation takes place after an intervention has been completed. If this mistake is made, it will generally lead to the conclusion that inadequate or inappropriate data were collected during the implementation of the intervention thereby prohibiting an adequate assessment of its effectiveness.

Table 7.2 The logical framework indicating project monitoring. Logical framework (as shown in Table 6.2) with boxes for monitoring highlighted

Narrative Summary (NS)	Verifiable Indicators (OVI)	Means of Verification (MoV)	Important Assumptions
Goal:			
Purpose:			
Outputs:			
1.			
2.			
3.			
4.			
5.			
Activities:			
1.1			
1.2			
:			
:			
2.1			
2.2			
:			
:			
3.1			
3.2			
:			
:			
:			
:			

Data Analysis and Reporting

It is important to give as much attention to how data are to be analysed and reported as it is to give to their specification and collection. Data are only of as much value as the uses to which they are put—unless they are converted into information and unless this information is employed to provide evidence in support of the decision-making process, data are worthless.

Exception Reporting Systems

Conventional analysis and reporting systems can give too little attention to this. They may generate large tabular formats (essentially turning data into more data) which require further analysis and/or interpretation which will be beyond the time availability of end-user decision-makers; or they may employ esoteric graphical

Table 7.3 The logical framework indicating project evaluation. Logical framework (as shown in Table 6.2) with boxes for evaluation highlighted

Narrative Summary (NS)	Verifiable Indicators (OVI)	Means of Verification (MoV)	Important Assumptions
Goal:			
Purpose:			
Outputs:			
1.			
2.			
3.			
4.			
5.			
Activities:			
1.1			
1.2			
:			
:			
2.1			
2.2			
:			
:			
3.1			
3.2			
:			
:			
:			
:			

representations which draw out features of interest only to statistical specialists rather than to lay information users.

Historically, information users from scientific or academic backgrounds have been primarily interested in the norm—measures of centrality and the spread of distributions around the centre. Decision-makers from a management or planning context will more usually be interested in *exceptions*—those management units (health districts or health facilities) that operate well above or well below the norm. The stronger units will call for special interest as they may be implementing practices from which other units can learn, thereby improving their own performance (or they may be a result of special characteristics of the unit and/or its environmental context). The weaker units will call for special attention as they may have the potential to improve their performance; or again 'poor' indicators may be a reflection of the special characteristics of the unit and/or its environment, in which case adaptations or additional provisions may be needed.

To convert raw data into information and evidence that meets the requirement of such decision-making contexts necessitates the development and use of *exception reporting systems*. These are reporting systems designed to alert decision-makers to units that lie outside of the norm.

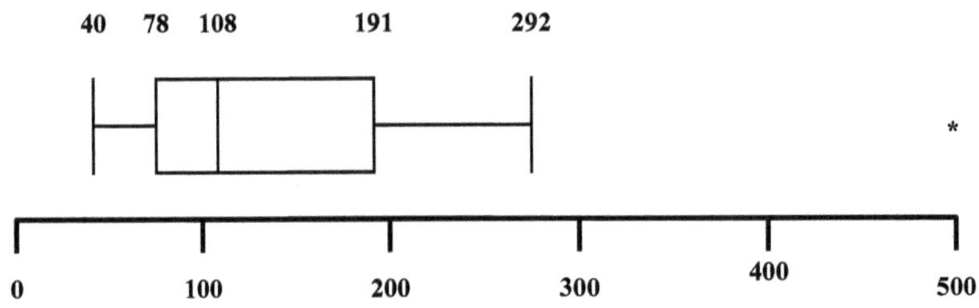

Fig. 7.1 Box-and-Whisker plot: Utilisation of PHS facilities—Gboko LGA, Benue State, Nigeria

Exploratory Data Analysis

Recent decades have seen the emergence of a set of techniques of data analysis and presentation which are more suited to such contexts. They are generically referred to as *Exploratory Data Analysis* approaches. Illustrative of such approaches is the *box plot* which is used in place of the more conventional histogram. The box plot is also called a box-and-whisker plot, as the core of the plot is a box with two whiskers, respectively, extending above and below. To draw a box plot (or box-and-whisker plot), the data is put in order of magnitude and divided into four equal parts known as quartiles. The midpoint of the data, the boundary between the second and third quartiles, is the measure of centrality generally called the median. A box is drawn from the respective outer edges of the second and third quartiles with the median indicated by a line within the box. To situate the whiskers, a distance of 1.5 times the interquartile range (or midspread—being the length of the box between the outer edges of the second and third quartiles) is calculated. The whisker is drawn at the nearest value inwards towards the box (being the next lowest or next highest at the respective ends). Any individual data values lying beyond the upper or lower whiskers are indicated explicitly. An example of a box plot is shown in Fig. 7.1. More details of its construction can be seen in a standard text such as Elliott and Marsh (2008).

In addition to its visual advantages over the conventional histogram, the box plot can be used to show the comparative distribution of an indicator across unit groupings—known as a multiple box plot. If, for example, the indicator of interest is the number of households in a community with access to a safe water supply, individual box plots for districts can be drawn showing the distribution of communities according to this indicator for individual districts. The box plots for each district within a region can then be laid alongside each other providing a composite regional picture (Fig. 7.2).

Information Flows to Decision-Makers

The purpose of employing a visual representation is to enhance the ease with which information can be conveyed to data users. An accompanying narrative can be used to draw out the critical issues, but this should not be a repetitive listing of general

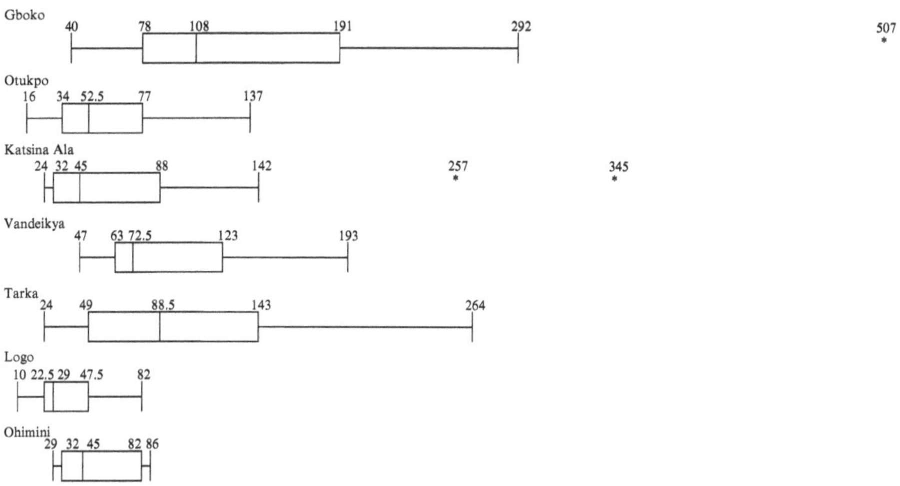

Fig. 7.2 Multiple box-and-Whisker plot: Utilisation of PHC facilities—all Benue Health Fund LGAs, Benue State, Nigeria

features. To aid the immediacy of interpretation, it is now a frequent procedure to employ a *traffic light system*. This can be particularly helpful where a set of multiple core indicators is being reported.

As an example of a traffic light system for use at the district level, individual health units will be listed with a column for each of the core indicators. Those lying within the main body of values (say, between the whiskers of the box plot) will be uncoloured. Those lying just within the poor performing area (just outside of the lower whisker) will be shown in amber; those lying well outside the poor performing area will be shown in red. Any units lying outside of the whisker at the other end (the well-performing area) will be shown in green.

Information Feedback to Data Providers

Of equal importance to the flow of information to decision-makers is the flow of information to data providers. We have already highlighted the importance of feedback as a means of ensuring that data providers are aware of the importance of maintaining a regular flow of reliable data. But beyond this feedback is vital to enable them to compare their own performance with that of similar units. However, this should be undertaken in a supportive non-judgemental way emphasising that performance of units may vary because of differing contexts—resourcing (particularly human resourcing), characteristics of the population being served, the complexity of the local terrain, etc. If it is felt by staff within units that they are being judged against their peers in the form of a league table, they may be encouraged to act perversely. They may falsify data to ensure a high score; or they may neglect areas of activity that are not captured within the set of core indicators, not withstanding its intrinsic local importance. Financial rewards have been used in a number of health systems to encourage higher levels of reporting or to reward good performance. Such measures should only be introduced if accompanied by strong supportive supervision (for which there is never a substitute), otherwise similar perverse consequences may ensue.

Further Discussion

In this chapter, we have looked briefly at the critical role that measurement can play in the planning and management of decentralised health services. We have cautioned against the natural tendency to over-collection and over-reporting of data, suggesting that agreement on a core set of indicators can ensure that both collection and reporting are purposeful and that through this confidence in the information production system is maintained. We have suggested that use of a logical framework (or a similar representational device) at the planning stage can facilitate the maintenance of focus. We have illustrated some approaches to data analysis and presentation which can enhance the accuracy with which information is relayed. This will strengthen its use as evidence within the decision-making process.

None of this should be taken prescriptively. There is no blueprint or recipe for evidence-based decision-making within decentralised health-care systems. The individuality of health systems which prompts the adoption of decentralised decision-making processes should also prompt the development and adoption of locally crafted information systems. Global initiatives, such as the achievement of the Millennium Development Goals, may provide some common starting points. But they cannot be translated slavishly down to the local level. An important and an essential characteristic of decentralised health-care systems is that they do not eliminate the necessary functions of higher (national and regional) levels within the system. Rather, they provide them with an essential focus (and relieve them from inappropriately and wastefully attempting to micro-manage localities). This essential focus is the determination of broad policy and the setting of parameters for longer term planning. If these functions are being effectively undertaken, it will be reflected in the district level health information systems. It is not inappropriate (indeed it may be taken as sign of the successful operation of the decentralised system) for regions and even districts themselves to identify their own core indicators to complement those that are required for national reporting.

There are also a number of constraining issues that should be taken into account when developing decentralised information systems. Not least of these are the availability and deployment of technical analytic skills and judicious employment of new technology. It is unlikely that individual districts will enjoy the luxury of a fully trained statistician. But if such skills are available at a regional level the supervisory system, augmented by regular regional level meetings focussing on health information, can be exploited to ensure that districts are recording data accurately and employing them themselves to support evidence-based decisions.

It is tempting to see computerisation as a panacea. But new technology is fraught with as many dangers as those that it overcomes. Ill-considered or overhasty moves to computerisation have regularly dismantled functioning manual systems leaving very little in their place. A frequent mistake is to attempt to revise the content of information systems simultaneously to their computerisation. Teething technical problems (which should be seen as inevitable and unavoidable) can destroy confidence in the whole information system and lead to a spiral of decline. However, if carefully and thoughtfully introduced, innovative use of widespread technological facilities, such as the mobile telephone network, can provide a valuable cog in the machinery of recording and reporting.

Recommended Reading

Marsh, C. (1988). *Exploring data—An introduction to data analysis for social scientists*. Cambridge: Polity.

Kielmann, A., Janovsky, K., & Annett, H. (1991). *Assessing district health needs, services and systems*. London: The Macmillan Press in conjunction with AMREF and GTZ.

A training manual which includes a range of survey instruments for the collection of data on health needs, health resources and the operation of health systems at the district level.

PAHO Special Group for Health Analysis. (2001). Health indicators: Building blocks for health situation analysis. *Epidemiological Bulletin, 22*(4), 1–5. Available at: http://www.who.int/management/district/assessment/HealthIndicatorsBuildingBlocksHealthSituationAnalysis.pdf

A good introduction and discussion of Health Indicators. Describes the PAHO/WHO Core Health Data Initiative and provides examples of National Basic Indicators from a range of Latin American countries.

Klassen, W., & Moynnihan, M. (2005). *Information: Its collection and use throughout the Project Cycle*. Network Learning: Amsterdam. Available at: http://www.who.int/management/collectinginformation.pdf

Provides a general discussion of the importance of good information within the planning process and moves through the planning cycle showing how information is fed into the Project Logical Framework.

References

Elliott, J., & Marsh, C. (2008). *Exploring data—An introduction to data analysis for social scientists*. Cambridge: Polity.

Parkinson J. (2012). *Establishing a core set of national, sustainable mental health indicators for children and young people in Scotland: Final Report*. NHS Health Scotland. Available at: http://www.healthscotland.com/uploads/documents/18751-C&YP%20Mental%20Health%20Indicators%20FINAL%20Report.pdf

Rigby, M., Köhler, L. (eds) (2002). *Child health indicators of life and development (CHILD): Report to the European Commission*. Centre for Health Planning and Management, Keele, UK, for European Commission Health and Consumer Protection Directorate. Available at: http://www.europa.eu.int/comm/health/ph/programmes/monitor/fp_monitoring_2000_frep_08_en.pdf

Chapter 8
Impact of Decentralization on Health Systems: Existing Evidence

Mario S. de Leon

Abstract This chapter helps the reader to understand and decide whether to accept or reject some of the evidence available and analysed on the impact of decentralization in health systems worldwide. This chapter also contributes to develop the reader's thinking about how to critically analyse some of the evidence identified, gathered and presented on the impact outcomes of decentralization in health systems, the variety and complexity of the decentralization effects and its institutional, political, legal, managerial, administrative and fiscal process, as well as its overall transformative aim. The reader analyses examples of the main objectives/outcomes of decentralization according to previous research carried out with that purpose. Hence, the existing evidence on decentralization outcomes expected/unexpected and achieved/unachieved. Whether or not, both kinds of decentralization paradigms (i.e. multi-sectoral and sectoral-wide or narrow approaches) would have effectively resolved or unresolved, improved or worsened and enhanced or reduced somehow those processes, changes, priorities, problems and needs at the different levels of implementation, structures and resources existing in the health system or sector in different countries.

After Reading This Chapter, the Reader Will Be Able to

- *Determine some of the features of the appraisal approaches presented in this chapter (i.e. Critical Comparative Literature Review (CLR) and Evidence Based Research (EBR)), to assess some of the evidence available, whether it has enough robustness (validity and generalisability) or not on the impact outcomes of decentralization as either multi-sectoral or sectoral process aimed to health systems/sectors.*

M.S. de Leon (✉)
Centre for the Study of Conflict, Power and Violence (CEDESCPV) in Europe, London, UK
e-mail: deleonsergio@hotmail.com

K. Regmi (ed.), *Decentralizing Health Services: A Global Perspective*,
DOI 10.1007/978-1-4614-9071-5_8,

- *Understand the kinds of impact outcomes and effects amongst some of the different components of the health systems provided through specific CLR and EBR examples, which are related to the eight main objectives of decentralization impact on health systems.*
- *To identify the pros and cons of achieving or not the main eight objectives of decentralization according to some of the CLR and EBR issues found. Likewise, what are the reasons these objectives can become either positive or negative outcomes overall.*

Introduction

There are two related conceptual paradigms for the study of decentralization affecting any health system structure and functioning (Asfaw et al. 2007; Jiménez-Rubio 2010). Both are based on how widely or narrowly decentralization is applied amongst institutionalised and organised sectors of society in different low-, middle- and high-income countries worldwide.

In the first paradigm, decentralization is a wide multi-sectoral process or aim, which is implemented to modify, change or transform legal, political, administrative, managerial, economic and fiscal policies and institutions of the government (UNDP 1999; WB 2001). Also, other political, economic and social sectors of society may simultaneously or not be modified, changed or transformed. Decentralization is established progressively by a rationale of conceptual and comprehensive planning to produce the changes in the middle and long run. Within the first paradigm, decentralization efforts also modify or enhance codes, norms, regulations, structures, infrastructure, resources and procedures for their implementation and development seeking to improve the quality, effectiveness and efficiency of services provided (Evans 2002; Erlandsen 2007).

In the second paradigm, decentralization is a wide or narrow focused or specific and mostly sectoral process or aim, which is implemented and concentrated on reforming different parts of the structure and functions of a specific institutional sector structure or social service provision, (e.g. the health sector, its different tiers and components) (Docteur and Oxley 2003; Burau and Blank 2006). Decentralization within this paradigm touches the three infrastructural, financial and organisational levels of the health services, (primary, secondary and tertiary). The second paradigm (sectoral decentralization) is the most important part addressed by this chapter, which, simultaneously acknowledges the interconnection between both paradigms and the fact that the second paradigm is usually part of and depends on the first one. For instance, it usually depends on general strategic policy planning, financial allocation and transfers and labour force pension schemes, etc.

Both kinds of decentralization paradigms are institutionally or organisationally planned and carried out by the Ministry of Health (MOH) and the government sector, in contractual or another kind of combined partnerships between statutory, civil and voluntary and/or private sectors (Berger and Messer 2002; Eggleston 2009).

Table 8.1 Example of the evidence-based research found on IITE

Critical appraisal carried out by I. Joumard, C. Andre and C. Nicq (2010). 'Health care systems: efficiency and institutions'. OECD Economics Department Working Papers. No. 769. OECD Publishing, as source example of Improved Institutional and Technical Efficiency (IITE).
Conclusions and Recommendations
• The paper concludes that big bang reforms (sudden, quick and extended) in the healthcare system are not effective or may cause more harm than benefit.
• Efficiency in healthcare spending is better understood by estimating the contribution of healthcare efficient spending and preventing measures to extend and enhance life expectancy and quality of life, taking into account socio-economic factors and lifestyle.
• It is important to consider the policy framework and cost-effectiveness relies upon a coherent policy framework.
• Adopt best policy practices and borrow the most appropriate elements from other systems.
• Further work is needed on pharmaceutical sector, coordination of care and sick leaves as there is no solid analysis.
• Existing indicators may need to be refined in the health insurance markets and for out-of-pocket payments.
• Overall measuring performance is challenging and full potential efficiency gains are underestimated.

Also, both paradigms are designed, implemented and evaluated using diverse standard approaches, methodologies and conceptual frameworks according to specific ideological, political, conceptual, technical, financial and economic agendas (i.e. techno-bureaucratic systems, market mechanisms and democratic participative approaches) (Cole 1999; Green 2007; de Leon 2010). Hence, the focus of this chapter is:

First, to analyse critically and comparatively some key elements of decentralization. It is mainly done as the second paradigm and within the health sector. Second, to apply two methodologies Critical Comparative Literature Review with 48 synthesised examples (24 positive and 24 negative) and Evidence-Based Research (EBR) with 8 examples summarised presenting the recommendations and conclusions (Tables 8.1–8.8). These examples demonstrate the positive and negative interrelationships and impact outcomes produced by decentralization upon the different components and aspects of health systems in the short, middle and long run worldwide. Third, to discuss some of the most important positive and negative (sometimes undefined, undetermined or neutral) impact outcomes that decentralization has produced amongst different health systems.

Health Decentralization: Focus and Scope of Impact Outcomes

In the last 20 years, there have been institutional, political and social national and international fora, technical meetings and workshops, political debates and research studies in favour or against its implementation and foreseen outcomes (Nieves and

Table 8.2 Example of evidence-based research on IAEE

Critical appraisal carried out by Weatherly, H. et al. (2010). 'Financial Integration Across Community and Social Care: Evidence Review'. Scottish Government Social Research, as source example of Increased Allocative Efficiency and Expenditure (IAEE).
Conclusions and Recommendations
• It is difficult to determine which factors are critical to success of IRFs (Integrated Resource Frameworks).
• The study found inclusiveness, inter-agency approach and flexibility as amongst the factors
• Overall evidence on cost-effectiveness is limited.
• Gaps in the study related to the quality of studies, the outcomes assessed and reporting of the model of financial integration.
• There is a strong need for data collection. Randomised control trials (CTs) can be a key source for evidence collection, but few studies use this method.
• Analysis of integration costs, which might be high, and evaluation are needed.
• The report draws out lessons to be learnt in linking the varied sources of money spent on populations, many of whom have complex needs.
• Empirical evaluations identified the effectiveness and costs of the IRMs and barriers to implementing them.
• Full structural integration of healthcare or health and social care is rare, and there is little evidence to suggest that this approach is necessary or sufficient to achieve successful partnership working.

Table 8.3 Example of evidence-based research on ELTLG

Critical appraisal carried out by Bossert, T. J. and J. C. Beavais (2002) 'Decentralization of health systems in Ghana, Zambia and Uganda and the Philippines: a comparative analysis of decision space' in Health Planning and Policy. 17(1):14–31, as source example of Empowering Lower Tiers of Local Governments (ELTLG).
Conclusions and Recommendations
• It is possible to draw preliminary conclusions about the countries experiences with decentralization against several categories.
• Performance evaluation is recommended.
• The research also concludes that following the extensive review of material and comparative data that there is insufficient evidence to assess the impact of decentralization on the population using the health system as this is the most important factor.
• However the research identifies a number of challenges for future research as factors related to spending, local decision-making, sector performance and expenditure are complex variables.

La Forgia 2000; Gragnolati and Marini 2003). Decentralization is still now one of the most controversial policy issues in international development (Colombo and Tapay 2004; Braga de Macedo et al. 2009). Likewise, according to WHO (2009), in the last 20 years more than 80 % of the countries worldwide had experienced and experimented somehow with either one of both decentralization paradigms explained above (Work and UNDP/BDP 2002; Docteur and Oxley 2003). It has been implemented throughout North America, Latin America, Europe, Asia, Australasia and Africa. Furthermore, according to Campbell (2003) and Braga de Macedo et al. (2009), at the start of the 2000s and after more than 20 years of

Table 8.4 Example of evidence-based research on IANHP

Critical appraisal carried out by Walshe, K. and T. Rundall (2001) 'Evidence-based management: from Theory to practice in Healthcare. The Milibank Quarterly, 79(3): 429-457', as source example of Increasing the Adoption of New Ways/Approaches of Health Service Provision (IANHP).
Conclusions and Recommendations
• An agenda for action to promote evidence-based practice.
• The needs to make managers more aware of research practice towards long-term managerial involvement in research.
• Government-led and system-wide changes and increased investment.
• Using evidence in decision-making by healthcare managers and policymakers.
• There is scope for the much better use of evidence.
• Managerial and clinical practice are very different, so evidence-based management in healthcare is unlikely to follow the established clinical model.
• If evidence is to play a greater role in how managers make decisions, managers need to be more aware of research. Implementation of evidence-based practices will require government and system-based support.
• It concludes that there is wide variation and the evidence is ambiguous.

Table 8.5 Example of evidence-based research on the impact of IHSDHSD

Critical appraisal carried out by MacMillan, R. (2010). 'The third sector delivering public services: an evidence review'. Third Sector Research Centre; 'Working Paper 20', as source example of Innovating the Health Service Delivery (IHSD).
Conclusions and Recommendations
• There are a number of key research gaps.
• How commissioning models, co-production and personalisation impact the third sector is not known, and inter-organisational responses like collaborations need further research as organisations are complex structure.
• There is a degree of polarisation with national versus local and issues around sustainability and resilience impacts upon organisational abilities to participate in commissioning.
• The policy arena is open and emerging in real time. The question – whether the third sector is an alternative provider of public services or whether recent experience has placed the sector in a different position – is open to further research.

decentralization, national and local governments/ authorities worldwide have spent between 10 and 50 % of total revenues generated by themselves implementing the modalities of health decentralization, although soft loans have been given by the IFIs and the international aid community worldwide supporting that purpose as well (Campbell 2003; Braga de Macedo et al. 2009).

Nevertheless, the ideological contents, rationale and objectives of health decentralization policies have mostly been oriented towards techno-bureaucratic systems approaches (TBSA) and market mechanism approaches (MMA) (Cole 1999; Green 2007; de Leon 2010). In many cases a critical analysis of the two approaches mentioned above, both central governments and private sectors have simultaneously been the main authorities/responsible to implement and develop health decentralization

Table 8.6 Example of evidence-based research on the impact of EMAHS

Critical appraisal carried out by L. S. Ramiro, F. A. Castillo, T. Tan-Torres, C. E. Torres, J. G. Tayag, R. G. Talampas and L. Hawken (2001) 'Community participation in local health boards in a decentralized setting: cases from the Philippines. Health Policy Planning. 16(suppl 2): 61-69', as source example of Enhancing the Mechanisms of Accountability in the Health System (EMAHS).

Conclusions and Recommendations

- Functioning LCBs tended to score better on the following variables: awareness of devolution, empowerment, participation, involvement and overall satisfaction with health services.
- The study was also able to break down key variables related to participation, for example, the involvement of other sectors in the health sector tended to improve the perception of participation.
- In functioning LCBs, the role of health officers was more active especially around decision-making.
- The study was able to identify the determinants of popular participation as being: awareness, capacity to influence decisions and opportunity to participate.
- These findings were central to the hypothesis.
- Using a range of perception-based indicators, the study was able to draw clear conclusions about level, degree and nature of participation in relation to the responsiveness and accountability of the system.
- The study was able to recommend the need for broader community participation in relation to breaking down political, sociocultural, psychological and financial barriers.

Table 8.7 Example of evidence-based research on the impact of RQHS

Critical appraisal carried out by Lagarde M., Haines, A. and Palmer, N. (2007). Conditional Cash Transfers for Improving Uptake of Health Interventions in Low- and Middle-Income Countries: A Systematic Review; JAMA. 298(16):1900–1910, as source example of Raising the Quality of Health Services (RQHS).

Conclusions and Recommendations

- While certain aspects are improved by using cash transfers such as use of healthcare, improving nutrition and anthropometric behaviour, outcomes and preventative behaviours, the overall effect on the health status is less clear.
- This highlights the importance on effective health programmes for demand-side programmes.
- The study recommends further research to investigate the impact on conditional cash transfers in different settings and to assess the pathways by which effects are achieved.
- Further evaluation is needed for low-income countries where means testing is more difficult.
- This review of evidence from 6 conditional cash transfer programmes reveals a reasonably consistent picture of the effects of such programmes on health-related behaviours and, to some extent, outcomes.
- These types of demand-side strategies seem successful in increasing use of health services and improving nutritional and anthropometric outcomes and preventive behaviours.
- However, their overall effect on health status remains less clear.
- This highlights the importance of a focus on the supply of adequate and effective health services for demand-side programmes such as these to have a more reliable effect on health outcomes.

Table 8.8 Example of evidence-based research on the impact of IEAHS

Critical appraisal carried out by Crook, R. C. (2003). Decentralization and poverty reduction in Africa: the politics of local–central relations. Public Administration Development, 23: 77–88, as source example of Increasing Equity and Accessibility of Health Services (IEAHS).
Conclusions and Recommendations
• The lack of data affects the quality of comparative and systematic review.
• The research found that administrative and political decentralization is affected by local-central relation and the regime context.
• That it is very much influenced by the ideological conviction of central political authorities towards policy reduction. Decentralization has not empowered challenges to local elites.
• It is likely that decentralization will empower any real challenge to local elites who are resistant to or uninterested in development of pro-poor policies, except possibly South Africa if the regime sees a political advantage in using local government for this purpose.
• On the contrary, in most of the African cases, 'elite capture' of local power structures has been facilitated by the desire of ruling elites to create and sustain power bases in the countryside.
• Popular perceptions of the logic of patronage politics reinforce this outcome. Even where the interests of underprivileged groups and of the rural poor have achieved some representation through democratic decentralization, accountability mechanisms are in general not strong enough to ensure that these interests are represented effectively in policymaking.
• These are the political realities, which have a shaping influence on the outcomes of decentralization policies in Africa.
• Any prospect of using decentralised governance to develop more pro-poor policies must depend upon a real effort being undertaken to strengthen and broaden accountability mechanisms, both horizontal and vertical, at both local and national levels.

as well as the main beneficiaries of its implementation, adoption and impact outcomes (Cole 1999; de Leon 2010). Thus, there have been very few examples about the levels of success of democratic participative process approaches (DPA), their grassroots and horizontal organisational structures and the evidence of their participation in decision-making, governance, accountability and so on, as overall impact outcomes on health systems through health decentralization efforts worldwide (Cole 1999; Schou 2003; de Leon 2010).

Decentralization and Health Systems

WHO/HSP (2001) has stated that a health system includes all actors, institutions and resources that undertake health actions. A health action is defined as the primary intent to improve health in a comprehensively manner. Hence, although the defining goal of a health system is to improve the population's health, there are other intrinsic (necessary, related and complementary) goals for which a health system must be responsive to the population it serves (WHO/HSP 2001; WHO 2007). These intrinsic goals are determined by the way and the environment in which people are treated. Also, by ensuring that the financial burden of paying for health services is fairly distributed across households and most or all of the population sectors.

Policymakers and populations are vitally concerned about their health systems, how they are performing and where, what and how they can be improved (WHO 2007, 2009). Many different types of reforms and policies have been aimed at improving the performance of health systems. They both have been introduced over the last decades worldwide and at all levels of development. Yet, the evidence about what works and what does not is limited and mixed, and the debate about appropriate health systems development is often led more by ideology than by evidence (WHO 2007, 2009; Wendt 2009).

Meanwhile, there are many studies on the decentralization impact on health systems and health status, focused on the aim and the objective outcomes of it (see Tables 8.1–8.8). Those studies applied different methods to identify and establish the evidence on the relationships between health decentralization impact outcomes and their best indicators. Nevertheless, it is not easy to measure the array of impacts that health decentralization has on health systems (e.g. in planning decision-making and implementation of infrastructure, resources and services) and thus the effects on the health status of populations. The main aim of decentralization in the health sector is to modify the design or content, the implementation and the function of policies, planning and financing norms, structures, procedures, performances/roles and results-outcomes. Therefore, all these elements should be transformed by decentralization to a more effectively, efficiently, fairly/equitably and accountably redefined, restructured and redeveloped core content of any health system (Cole 1999; Green 2007; de Leon 2010).

Improving Institutional and Technical Efficiency

Improved Institutional and Technical Efficiency (IITE) in a health system has been implemented reorganising bureaucracies, their tasks, functions and interactions. Public/private health services have been working in partnerships, established under a single or more decision-making authorities. Stakeholders, beneficiaries and clients/users have been involved in seeking more effectively and efficiently public health interventions through decentralised policies and initiatives (Or 2000; Robalino et al. 2001; Collins and Green 1993)

Positive CLR Evidence on the Impact of IITE

Here in three bullet points, the reader has some examples summarised applying CLR on Improved Institutional and Technical Efficiency (IITE) in the last 20 years:

- Imposition of greater 'cost-consciousness policies' to reduce expenditures have brought up 'creative ideas' throughout tier levels of government/authority (Colombo and Tapay 2004).
- The reconceptualisation of health planning strategies has been focussed on seeking overall effectiveness and efficiency, to implement health packages (Cutler 2002; Robalino et al. 2001).

- Quality assurance procedures have created environmental, technological and logistic conditions to enhance effectiveness and efficiency levels in health services (Ennis 2006; Hussey et al. 2009).

Negative CLR Evidence on the Impact of IITE

Here in three bullet points, the reader has some negative examples summarised on Improved Institutional and Technical Efficiency (IITE) in the last 20 years:

- The implementation of health decentralization policies has not clearly been communicated regarding its intensions, aims and objectives (Goetz and Gaventa 2001; WHO 2007).
- Users have not been provided with clear and efficient access to information to elicit appropriate collaborative responses to healthcare providers (Cornwall et al. 2000; Brinkerhoff 2004).
- Grants have been managed institutionally and technically in inefficient ways, creating setbacks in health service provision (Litvack et al. 1998; WB 2000).

Increasing Allocative Efficiency and Expenditure

The Increase in Allocative Efficiency and Expenditure has been achieved by consolidating budget allocations and expenditure targets through effective planning and implementation procedures by matching better the health services according to local preferences, by implementing proper assessments on priorities and needs fulfilled throughout timed cycles and by establishing health service packages aligned with programmed expenditure cycles (Goetz and Gaventa 2001; Cantarero and Pascual 2008).

Positive CLR Evidence on the Impact of IAEE

Here in three bullet points, the reader has some positive examples summarised on Increased Allocative Efficiency and Expenditure (IAEE) in the last 20 years:

- Stakeholders have effectively been involved discussing budget allocation in public health interventions at the local level (WB 2004; Jacobs et al. 2007).
- Expenditure allocation assessments in market-type relations (e.g. health insurance coverage) have been done through participative agreements with local populations (Gilson and Erasmus 2006; Erlandsen 2007).
- The funding allocation for innovative health packages have been conceptualised according to local/endemic priorities (Iwami and Petchey 2002; Brinkerhoff 2004).

Negative CLR Evidence on the Impact of IAEE

Here in three bullet points, the reader has some negative examples summarised on Increased Allocative Efficiency and Expenditure (IAEE) in the last 20 years:

- Public debts have endangered subnational economies, augmenting inequalities between and within regions (Macrae et al. 1996; Medved et al. 2005).
- Responsibility mismatches have frequently been found regarding revenue-raising/spending decisions between authorities (Craig et al. 2008; Mason and Goddard 2009).
- Conflicts have lacked enough leverage to elicit solutions for matching funds for underfunded health services (Smith 2008; Wagstaff 2009).

Empowering Lower Tiers of Local Governments (ELTLG)

The Empowerment of Lower Tiers of Local Governments (ELTLG) has been achieved through a more active local users'/customers' participation in decision-making processes, organised in representational groups or structures. ELTLG has also been achieved through transferring, establishing, enabling and improving the technical skills, administrative and managerial capabilities and good governance criteria to those local authorities and populations involved (PAHO 2004; Stegarescu 2005; Green 2007; de Leon 2010).

Positive CLR Evidence on the Impact of ELTLG

Here in three bullet points, the reader has some positive examples summarised on the Empowerment of Lower Tiers of Local Governments (ELTLG) in the last 20 years:

- Proper information exchanges have been established between health service providers and consumers in some countries (Belshaw 2000; Habibi et al. 2003; PAHO 2004).
- Accountability has been integrated beyond the mainstream bureaucratic and human resource realms (Lowensen et al. 2004; Sohani et al. 2005).
- Devolution has been successful combining capacity-building initiatives, authority functions and shared responsibilities at the local level (Crook and Manor 1998; Heller 2001).

Negative CLR Evidence on the Impact of ELTLG

Here in three bullet points, the reader has some negative examples summarised on Empowerment of Lower Tiers of Local Governments (ELTLG) in the last 20 years:

- Decentralization has increased dependencies and inequities in authority amongst lower government tiers at the subnational level (Pérez et al. 1995; Bach et al. 2009).

- Central political agendas have undermined local authorities, staff motivation and social accountability (Okuonzi and Macrae 1995; De Looper and Lafortune 2009).
- Organisational gaps have become standard issues, which decentralization not always can overcome (Smithson 1995; Bossuyt and Gould 2000).

Increasing the Adoption of New Ways/Approaches of Health Service Provision

The Increase in the Adoption of New Ways/Approaches of Health Service Provision (IANHP) has been achieved by adapting and adopting health services to local situations and conditions, increasing the autonomy of local governments and institutions (e.g. delegation or devolution) through decentralization policies. Also, authority responsibilities have been aligned and coordinated to serve population catchment areas, when they have been within one health district and two separate local government authorities, or vice versa (Davies et al. 1999; Macintyre et al. 2001; Chew and Osborne 2008).

Positive CLR Evidence on the Impact of IANHP

Here in three bullet points, the reader has some positive examples summarised on the Increased Adoption of New Ways/Approaches of Health Service Provision (IANHP) in the last 20 years:

- The enhancement of health allied and non-allied professionals roles and responsibilities has been accomplished by more local participative monitoring and evaluation feedback (Cutler 2002; Chapman et al. 2006).
- The quality and extension of delegation processes have been key components for successful decentralization approaches (Richards et al. 2000; Davies et al. 1999).
- Long-term infrastructure and human resource initiatives have benefited economically, socially, epidemiologically and environmentally to local communities (Fulop et al. 2003; Chew and Osborne 2008).

Negative CLR Evidence on the Impact of IANHP

Here in three bullet points, the reader has some negative examples summarised on the Increased Adoption of New Ways/Approaches of Health Service Provision (IANHP) in the last 20 years:

- Devolution has sometimes lead health providers to respond to local preferences for curative rather than preventive healthcare services (Belshaw 2000; Goetz and Gaventa 2001; Burau and Blank 2006).

- Local authorities have invested and prioritised other service sectors; hence, health services have starved of resources (PAHO 2004; Scott-Samuel et al. 2006).
- The private sector often participated more into goal curative-oriented approaches, usually without regulations (Meuwissen 2002; Standing 2004).

Innovating the Health Service Delivery

Innovation the Health Service Delivery (IHSD) has been achieved by creating new conceptual and operative frameworks to integrate health system networks and deliver better services by improving and integrating health services, information systems, staff performance and training and institutional and social accountability mechanisms related to decisions made/taken. This multi-sectoral integration has usually been provided with requirements, sanctions and penalties, supported by regulations and laws (Cutler 2002; De Looper and Lafortune 2009; Ramsay et al. 2009).

Positive CLR Evidence on the Impact of IHSD

Here in three bullet points, the reader has some positive examples summarised on the Innovation of the Health Service Delivery (IHSD) in the last 20 years:

- Decentralization corrective measures have reinforced strict budget constraints, strong management, fiscal discipline and rigorous accountability in health sectors (Mills 1996; De Looper and Lafortune 2009).
- The IFIs have established monitoring and evaluation frameworks for collective management systems to appraise the outcomes of fiscal policies over social services (Loewenson 2000; Ramsay et al. 2009).
- Redistribution of resources through equity tax policies has been resolved through checks and balances mechanisms placed by the international aid community (Mills 1994; De Looper and Lafortune 2009).

Negative CLR Evidence on the Impact of IHSD

Here in three bullet points, the reader has some negative examples summarised on the Innovation of the Health Service Delivery (IHSD) in the last 20 years:

- Decentralization has transferred spending and revenue-raising authority, but the lack of administrative capacity has lead to wasting resources (Docteur and Oxley 2003; Erlandsen 2007).
- Tension between vertical and horizontal integration has been associated with centralised vertical programmes and hierarchical donor funding (World 2001, 2004; Hofmarcher et al. 2007).

- District health committees have been established; however, their participatory effectiveness is mixed, because of clientelism, corruption or disinterest in involvement (Cutler 2002; Wendt et al. 2009; de Leon 2010).

Enhancing the Mechanisms of Accountability in Health Systems

The Enhancement of the Mechanisms of Accountability in Health Systems (EMAHS) have been achieved by establishing and improving the accountability strategies and mechanisms when transforming health systems by including governmentwide anti-corruption campaigns, health sector reform programmes, fiscal strategic approaches, transparency networks, etc. Accountability is still in constant construction and has been a permanent struggle for the grassroots movements. It has also been redefined and restructured to be more open, participative, horizontal, pluralistic and transparent (Cornwall et al. 2000; Heller 2001; Brinkerhoff 2004).

Positive CLR Evidence on the Impact of EMAHS

Here in three bullet points, the reader has some positive examples summarised on the Enhancement of the Mechanisms of Accountability in the Health System (EMAHS) in the last 20 years:

- Financial accountability has been developed to track down and report the allocation, disbursement and utilisation of financial resources (Brinkerhoff 2004; WHO 2009).
- Performance accountability has been implemented to assess the healthcare services, outputs and outcomes (Mills 1994).
- Political accountability has been created to ensure that elected governments deliver on electoral promises (Eaton 1998; Cornwall et al. 2000).

Negative CLR Evidence on the Impact of EMAHS

Here in three bullet points, the reader has some negative examples summarised on the Enhancement of the Mechanisms of Accountability in the Health System (EMAHS) in the last 20 years:

- Decentralization policies have not been properly analysed to ensure that authorities truly address the changing needs of people (Cole 1999; Brinkerhoff 2004).
- Local political and organisational capacity has not been strategically supported by central government authorities (Cornwall et al. 2000; Opwora et al. 2010).
- Some decentralization objectives have not been met yet in some countries due to structural constrains and political environments (Pérez et al. 1995; Brinkerhoff 2004).

Raising the Quality of Health Services

The Raise in the Quality of Health Services (RQHS) has been achieved by designing and enhancing the infrastructure and the provision of health services; by improving the quality and availability of physical, economic and human resources; by integrating the health services, the information systems and qualified staff/personnel; and, also in some countries, by utilising decentralization policies to open and extend the access to healthcare services for vulnerable groups, where the public health sector has tended to go towards privatisation under the banner of more efficient and effective health service provision (Goetz and Gaventa 2001; Gragnolati and Marini 2003; Gilson and Erasmus 2006).

Positive CLR Evidence on the Impact of RQHS

Here in three bullet points, the reader has some positive examples summarised on the Raise of the Quality of Health Services (RQHS) in the last 20 years:

- Analytical frameworks in developing countries have positively generalised those efficiency factors behind 'successful and unsuccessful' decentralization experiences (Braveman and Gruskin 2003).
- Managerial efficiency improvements have been critical to prepare staff for their new roles due to decentralization (Carmel and Harlock 2008).
- Responsiveness to local demands has been a very important determinant for any decentralization initiative to be successful (Bossert 1998; Nsibambi 1998).

Negative CLR Evidence on the Impact of RQHS

Here in three bullet points, the reader has some negative examples summarised on the Raise of the Quality of Health Services (RQHS) in the last 20 years:

- Confusion amongst decentralization objectives have been detected when applied in shifts in service mix, away from locally prioritised services and health needs (Gilson and Erasmus 2006).
- Devolution has lead health providers responding to local preferences, offering curative rather than preventive services (Bossert et. al. 2002; Heller 2001).
- Conflicts of interest have appeared when a health district works with two separate local authorities or vice versa, creating competition and health inequalities (Nsibambi 1998; Bossert et. al. 2002).

Increasing the Equity and Accessibility of Health Services

The Increase in the Equity and Accessibility of Health Services (IEAHS) has been achieved by allocating resources according to local needs, regarding the assessment of endemic profiles through local, national and international public health programmes. Also, by enabling local organisations to better meet the needs of particular groups; by providing equitable distribution of resources towards marginalised regions and groups, through cross-subsidy balancing mechanisms; and by developing alternative strategies and resources to tackle the health problems and better ways of organising institutional and non-institutional resources, amongst other initiatives (Bloom 2000; WHO 2000; Cutler 2002; Braveman and Gruskin 2003; Docteur and Oxley 2003; Schou 2003; Jacobs et al. 2007; De Looper and Lafortune 2009).

Positive CLR Evidence on the Impact of IEAHS

Here in three bullet points, the reader has some positive examples summarised on the Increase in Equity and Accessibility of Health Services (IEAHS) in the last 20 years:

- 'Horizontal inequity' has partially been solved by implementing subnational redistribution policies (WHO 2000; Braveman and Gruskin 2003).
- Results have also been mixed with programmes trying to reduce tax-base disparities amongst local governments (Bloom 2000; Cutler 2002).
- Some countries in transition have instituted programmes to reduce disparities in the per capita revenues of subnational governments (Jacobs et al. 2007; De Looper and Lafortune 2009).

Negative CLR Evidence on the Impact of IEAHS

Here in three bullet points, the reader has some negative examples summarised on the Increase in Equity and Accessibility of Health Services (IEAHS) in the last 20 years:

- Decentralization planning and implementation policies have not properly been identified or determined with regard to health priorities, according to health realities (Docteur and Oxley 2003; Schou 2003).
- The health services have expanded within a general culture of uncertainty, abuse of authority, opportunism, clientelism and patrimony (Bloom 2000; Braveman and Gruskin 2003; Jacobs et al. 2007).
- There has been a brain-drain problem or high inequalities in human health resources, which decentralization efforts have not be able to resolve (Jacobs et al. 2007; De Looper and Lafortune 2009).

Conclusion

From the 48 examples using CLR (24 positive and 24 negative) and the 8 examples showed in Tables 8.1–8.8 using EBR, the conclusions are the following: sectoral (heath) decentralization after more than 20 years since it became the flag of structural changes for the existing health systems and their administration and provision of social services worldwide still is ambiguous, not clearly determined and understood due to its complex holistic nature. On the one hand, from some of the positive examples on the decentralization impact on health systems and health and populations described in this chapter, it is possible to interpret some of the benefits brought to some countries and their health systems worldwide. On the other hand, from the negative examples, it is possible to interpret that this is a continuous process in the short, middle and long terms, in which negative outcomes have to be corrected in different ways as well as adapt and adopt more creative and proper ways to carry out the transformation based on the previous experiences of such decentralising processes to obtain better results overall. Thus, the impact of decentralization in health systems has to be constantly appraised, and conclusions and corrective approaches, strategies, actions and measures have to be taken to avoid as much as possible its negative outcomes. Nevertheless, all this rationale unfortunately will heavily depend on the political environment of the country, the political history, political decision-making processes, the prevalent institutional and organisational culture, socio-economic and ethnic problems and inequities, corruption and so on.

Further Analytical and Reflective Discussion/Exercise with Questions

1. What are your own conclusions over the negative/positive evidence on the impact of health decentralization upon health systems worldwide after reading this chapter? Provide your opinion with 3 positive and 3 negative examples.
2. Do you think that is very important to continue implementing health decentralization worldwide? If you think affirmatively, explain why? If you think negatively, explain why?
3. Assume you are a health planner and you need to further improve (more efficiently and effectively) the impact of the eight main objectives of health decentralization. What would you do? (Write a couple of pages mapping your ideas based on the information provided by this chapter, the recommended readings below and a chosen country by yourself, which will provide you with a setting or context.)

Recommended Reading

The first reading below is a study which examines whether decentralization has improved health system performance and presents an example from a middle-income country at the subnational level.

1. Atkinson, S., & Haran, D. (2004, November). Back to basics: Does decentralization improve health system performance? Evidence from Ceará in north-east Brazil. *Bulletin of the World Health Organization, 82*(11). http://www.scielosp.org/pdf/bwho/v82n11/v82n11a06.pdf

The second reading below is a study which comparatively analyses the 'decision space' in two very different countries. There are few studies focused on this key topic to understand the dynamics and changes through a decentralization process.

2. Bossert, T., Bowser, D., & Amenyah, J. (2007). Is decentralization good for logistics systems? Evidence on essential medicine logistics in Ghana and Guatemala. *Health Policy and Planning, 22*, 73–82. http://heapol.oxfordjournals.org/content/22/2/73.full.pdf+html

The third reading below, presents the new tendencies in some European countries, on rethinking their decentralization process and adjusting their health systems to the elasticity and contraction of the regional and global market.

3. Saltman, R. B. (2008). Decentralization, re-centralization and future European health policy. *The European Journal of Public Health, 18*, 104–106 http://eurpub.oxfordjournals.org/content/18/2/104.full.pdf+html

References

Asfaw, A., Frohberg, K., James, K. S., & Jütting, J. (2007). Fiscal decentralization and health outcomes: empirical evidence from rural India. *Journal of Developing Areas, 41*, 17–35.

Bach, S., Blöchliger, H., Wallau, D. (2009). "The spending power of sub-central governments: A pilot study", *OECD Economic Department Working Papers*, No. 705, OECD, Paris.

Belshaw, D. (2000). Decentralised governance and poverty reduction: Relevant experience in Africa and Asia. In P. Collins (Ed.), *Applying public administration in development: Guideposts for the future* (pp. 93–113). Chichester: Wiley.

Berger, M., & Messer, J. (2002). Public financing of health expenditure, insurance, and health outcomes. *Applied Economics, 34*(17), 2105–2113.

Bloom, G. (2000). Equity in health in unequal societies: Towards health equity during rapid social change. IDS Working Paper 112. Institute of Development Studies.

Bossert, T. (1998). Analyzing the decentralization of health systems in developing countries: Decision space, innovation, and performance. *Social Science and Medicine, 47*, 1513–27.

Bossert, T., Larrañaga, O., & Meir, F. R. (2002). Decentralization of health systems in Latin America. *Pan American Journal of Public Health, 8*(1/2), 84–92.

Bossuyt, J., & Gould, J. (2000). *Decentralization and poverty reduction: Elaborating the linkages. Policy Management Brief 12*. Maastricht, Netherlands: European Centre for Development Policy Management.

Braga de Macedo, J., Oliveira, J, Rocha, B. (2009). "*Growth and Policy Complementarities: Are Complementary Reforms a "Luxury" for Developing Countries*?". Paper presented at IZA-FRDB Workshop on "Tracking Structural Reforms", University Bocconi, Milan

Braveman, P., & Gruskin, S. (2003). Defining equity in health. *Journal of Epidemiology and Community Health, 57*, 254–258.

Brinkerhoff, D. W. (2004). Accountability and health systems: Toward conceptual clarity and policy relevance. *Health Policy and Planning, 19*, 371–379.

Burau, V., & Blank, R. H. (2006). Comparing health policy: An assessment of typologies of health systems. *Journal of Comparative Policy Analysis, 8*(1), 63–76.

Campbell, T. (2003). *Decentralization and the rise of political participation in Latin American cities*. Pittsburgh: University of Pittsburgh Press.

Cantarero, D., & Pascual, M. (2008). Analysing the impact of fiscal decentralization on health outcomes: Empirical evidence from Spain. *Applied Economic Letters, 15*, 109–111.

Carmel, E., & Harlock, J. (2008). Instituting the 'third sector' as a governable terrain: Partnership, procurement and performance in the UK. *Policy and Politics, 36*(2), 155–71.

Chapman, T., Brown, J., Crow, R., & Ward, J. (2006). *Facing the future: A study of the impact of a changing funding environment on the voluntary and community sector in the North East of England.* Middlesbrough: Social Futures Institute, Teesside University. 2006.

Chew, C., & Osborne, S. P. (2008). Strategic positioning in U.K. Charities that provide public services: Implications of a new integrating model. *Public Money and Management, 28*(5), 283–90.

Cole, K. (1999). *Economy-environment-development-knowledge.* London, UK: Routledge.

Collins, C., & Green, A. T. (1993). Decentralization and primary health care in developing countries ten key questions. *Journal of Management in Medicine, 7*, 58–68.

Colombo, F., & Tapay, N. (2004). *Private health insurance in OECD countries: The benefits and costs for individuals and health systems* (OECD Health Working Papers, No. 15). Paris: OECD.

Cornwall, A., Lucas, H., & Pasteur, K. (2000). Accountability through participation: Developing workable partnership models in the health sector. *IDS Bulletin, 2000*, 31.

Craig, P., et al. (2008). Developing and evaluating complex interventions: The new Medical Research Council guidance. *BMJ, 337*, a1655.

Crook RC, Manor J (3 Dec, 1998). Democracy and decentralization in South Asia and West Africa: Participation, accountability and performance. *Business & Economics.* Cambridge University Press, p. 335

Cutler, D. M. (2002). Equality, efficiency and market fundamentals: The dynamics of International Medical-care Reform. *Journal of Economic Literature, 40*(3), 881–906.

Davies, H. T. O., Nutley, S. M., & Smith, P. C. (1999). What works? The role of evidence in public sector policy and practice. *Public Money and Management, 19*(1), 3–5.

de Leon, M. S. (2010). *Health decentralization and post-conflict: An evaluation framework.* Berlin, Germany: VDM Verland Dr. Muller GmbH & Co KG.

De Looper, M., Lafortune, G. (2009). Measuring disparities in health status and in access and use of health care in OECD countries. *OECD Health Working Papers, No. 43*, Directorate for Employment, Labour and Social Affairs, OECD, Paris.

Docteur, E., & Oxley, H. (2003). Health care systems: Lessons from the reform experience. *OECD Health Working Papers 9.* Paris: OECD.

Eaton, M. (1998). Political obstacles to decentralization in Argentina and the Philippines. Unpublished paper, presented at the September 1998 conference of the *Latin American Studies Association*, Chicago.

Eggleston, K. (2009). Provider payment incentives: International comparisons. *International Journal of Health Care Finance and Economics, 9*(2), 113–115.

Ennis, S. (2006). Competition in the provision of hospital services. *Journal of Competition Law and Policy, 8*(3), 153–247.

Erlandsen, E. (2007). "Improving the efficiency of health care spending: Selected evidence on hospital performance", *OECD Economics Department Working Papers*, No. 555, OECD, Paris.

Evans, D. B. (2002). The evolution of WHO's approach to health system performance assessment, Chapter 9. In *Measuring up: Improving Health System Performance in OECD Countries.* Paris: OECD.

Fulop, N., Allen, P., Clarke, A., & Black, N. (2003). From health technology assessment to research on the organisation and delivery of health services: Addressing the balance. *Health Policy, 63*(2), 155–165.

Gilson, L., & Erasmus, E. (2006). *Trust and accountability in health service delivery in South Africa.* Johannesburg: Centre for Health Policy, University of Witwatersrand South Africa.

Goetz, A.M., Gaventa, J. (2001). Bringing citizen voice and client focus into service delivery. IDS Working Paper 138.

Gragnolati, M., & Marini, A. (2003). Health and poverty in Guatemala. World Bank. *World Bank Policy Research.* Working Paper 2966, January. Washington, USA.

Green, A. (2007). *An introduction to health planning for developing health systems* (3rd ed.). Oxford, UK: Oxford University Press.

Habibi, N., Huang, C., Miranda, D., Murillo, V., Ranis, G., Sarkar, M., et al. (2003). Decentralization and human development in Argentina. *Journal of Human Development, 4*(1).

Heller, P. (2001). Moving the state: the politics of democratic decentralization in Kerala, South Africa and Porto Alegre. *Politics and Society, 29*(1), 131–163.

Hofmarcher, M. M., Oxley, H., Rusticelli, E. (2007). Improved health system performance through better care coordination. *OECD Health Working Paper,* No. 30.

Hussey, P. S., de Vries, H., Romely, J., Wang, M. C., Chen, S. S., Shekelle, P. G., et al. (2009). A systematic review of health care efficiency measures. *Health Services Research, 44*(3), 784–805.

Iwami, M., & Petchey, R. (2002). A Class act? Community-based organizations, health service decentralization and primary care development in Peru. Local Committees for Health Administration. *Journal of Public Health Medicine, 24,* 246–251.

Jacobs, B., Price, N., & Sam, S. O. (2007). A sustainability assessment of a health equity fund initiative in Cambodia. *The International Journal of Health Planning and Management, 22,* 183–203.

Jiménez-Rubio, D. (2010, November). *Is fiscal decentralization good for your health? Evidence from a panel of OECD countries* (HEDG Working Paper 10/30). York, UK: University of York.

Litvack, J. I., Ahmad, J., & Bird, R. (1998). *Rethinking decentralization in developing countries* (Sector studies series). Washington, DC: World Bank.

Loewenson, R. (2000). *Participation and accountability in health systems: The missing factor in equity?* (pp. 1–27). Harare: TARSC.

Lowensen, R., Rusike, I., Zulu, M. (2004). Assessing the impact of Health Centre Committees on health system performance and health resource allocation 2004, Equinet Discussion Paper 18.

Macintyre, S., Chalmers, I., Horton, R., & Smith, R. (2001). Using evidence to inform health policy: Case study. *British Medical Journal, 322,* 222–5.

Macrae, J., Zwi, A., & Gilson, L. (1996). A triple burden for health sector reform: 'post'-conflict rehabilitation in Uganda. *Social Science and Medicine, 42,* 1095–108.

Mason, A., & Goddard, M. (2009). Payment by results in mental health: A review of the International Literature and an Economic Assessment of the approach in the English NHS. *CHE Research Paper 50*, 71.

Medved, J., Nemec, J., Vítek, L. (2005) "Social health insurance and its failure in the Czech Republic and Slovakia: The Role of the State", *Prague Economic Papers,* 1.

Meuwissen, L. E. (2002). Problems of cost-recovery implementation in district healthcare: A case study from Niger. *Health Policy Plan, 17,* 304–313.

Mills, A. (1994). Decentralization and accountability in the health sector from an international perspective: What are the choices? *Public Administration and Development, 14,* 281–92.

Mills, A. (1996). Decentralization concepts and issues: A review. In A. Mills, P. Vaughan, D. Smith, & I. Tabibzadeh (Eds.), *Health system decentralization: Concepts and issues* (p. 1996). Geneva: World Health Organization.

Nieves, I., & La Forgia, G. M. (2000). *Large-scale government contracting of NGOs to extend basic health services to poor populations in Guatemala.* Washington: WB.

Nsibambi, A. (1998). *Decentralization and civil society in Uganda* (p. 154). London, UK: Fountain Publishers.

Okuonzi, S. A., & Macrae, J. (1995). Whose policy is it anyway? International and national influences on health policy development in Uganda. *Health Policy and Planning, 10,* 122–32.

Opwora, A., Kabare, M., Molyneux, S., & Goodman, C. (2010). Direct facility funding as a response to user fee reduction: Implementation and perceived impact among Kenyan health centres and dispensaries. *Health Policy and Planning, 2010*(25), 406–418.

Or, Z. (2000). *Determinants of health outcomes in industrialised countries: A pooled, cross-country, time-series analysis (OECD Economic Studies No. 30).* Paris: OECD.

Pan American Health Organization (2004). An integrated, multi-disease community based approach in the control of soil-transmitted worms in Brazil Washington, DC

Pérez, J., Alfiler, M. C., Victorian, M. (1995). Decentralization and health systems change: Managing transition dilemmas in the early years of devolution in the Philippines. Country report, World Health Organization (WHO), Decentralization and Health Systems Change Project

Ramsay, A., Fulop, N., & Edwards, N. (2009). The evidence base for vertical integration in health care. *Journal of Integrated Care, 17*, 3–12.
Richards, A., Carley, J., Jenkins-Clarke, S., & Richards, D. A. (2000). Skill-mix between nurses and doctors working in primary care-delegation or allocation? A review of the literature. *International Journal of Nursing Studies, 37*, 185–97.
Robalino, D. A., Picazo, O. F., & Voetberg, A. (2001). *Does fiscal decentralization improve health outcomes? Evidence from a crosscountry analysis (Policy Research Working Paper No. 2565).* Washington DC: World Bank.
Schou, A. (2003). 'Synthesis study on supporting decentralization and local government—Lessons Learned, Good Practices and Emerging Issues'. Report for the DAC Working Party on Aid Evaluation, OECD. [www.uneval.org/docs/DAC_EV(2003).3.doc].
Scott-Samuel, A., Ardern, K., & Birley, M. (2006). Assessing health impacts on a population. In D. Pencheon, C. Guest, D. Melzer, & J. A. Muir Gray (Eds.), *Oxford handbook of public health practice* (2nd ed., pp. 42–55). Oxford: Oxford University Press.
Smith, P. C., (2008). Market mechanisms and the use of health care resources. In *Achieving Better Value for money in Health Care,* OECD Health Policy Studies. OECD, Paris
Smithson, P. (1995). Quarts into pint jugs? The financial viability of health sector investment in low income countries. *Health Policy and Planning, 10*(Suppl.), 6–16.
Sohani, S. B., Borg, J., & Fox, J. (2005). *Managing a health facility: A handbook for committee members and facility staff* (2nd ed.). Kenya: Ministry of Health & Aga Khan Health Service.
Standing, H. (2004). *Understanding the 'demand side' in service delivery: definitions, frameworks and tools from the health sector.* Institute of Development Studies, University of Sussex.
Stegarescu, D. (2005). Public sector decentralization: Measurement concepts and recent international trends. *Fiscal Studies*, 301–333.
United Nations Development Project (1999). Decentralized governance monograph: A global sampling of experience" September 1999.
Wagstaff, A. (2009). Social health insurance versus tax-financed health systems—evidence from the OECD", *World Bank Policy Research Working Paper*, No. 4821
World Bank (WB). (2000). *World Development Report 1999/2000: Entering the 21st century.* Washington, DC: World Bank.
World Bank (2001). *Different forms of decentralization and rationale for decentralisation.* Electronic Website Washington D C. [Online October 2012] www1.worldbank.org/publicsector/decentralization/what.htm
World Bank (2004). Making services work for poor people. World Development Report 2004
Wendt, C. (2009). Mapping European Healthcare Systems: A comparative analysis of financing, service provision and access to healthcare. *Journal of European Social Policy, 19*(5), 432–45.
Wendt, C., Frisina, L., & Rothgang, H. (2009). Healthcare system types: A conceptual framework for comparison. *Social Policy and Administration, 43*(1), 70–90.
World Health Organisation. (2000). *The world health report (2000). Health systems: Improving performance.* Geneva: WHO.
World Health Organisation. (2007). *Everybody's business—strengthening health systems to improve health outcomes. WHO's Framework for Action.* Geneva: WHO.
World Health Organisation (2009). "Health Systems, Health and Wealth", WHO European Ministerial Conference on Health Systems, 25–27 June 2008, Tallinn, Estonia
World Health Organisation/Health Systems Performance (2001). Concepts and definitions. WHO Evidence for Health Policy. ~Electronic Webpage Geneva Switzerland, 2001. http://www.who.int/health-systems-performance/about.htm#What%20is%20a%20health%20 system?
Work, R. and UNDP/BDP (2002). 'The role of participation and partnership in decentralised governance: A brief synthesis of policy lessons and recommendations of Nine Country Case Studies on Service Delivery for the Poor' [www.undp.org/governance/ docsdecentral/participationandpartnershippdf.pdf].

Chapter 9
Participation in the New Public Health Landscape

Matthew Almond

Abstract The UK government's proposals for devolving power to local authorities and encouraging individuals to take more responsibility in these deliberations are changing the landscape of social and political decision-making and their responsiveness to the public. As a result there are major implications for public health in this process and how the public are consulted and involved and the challenges that they represent. The impact of this process will be explored in two ways. First, an exploration of what it means to be involved in decision-making through a discussion of participation, empowerment and agency. This raises questions about how the individual can be realistically involved and how the health professional's role can be faithful to the principles of facilitating change and enabling individuals to engage. Second, the section on theory into practice will examine how we can translate these ideas into practical guidance and action. It will explore what is the evidence base for community engagement and outline some examples of what action can be taken. Finally, series of questions are posed after each section to enable the reader to explore these issues and a number of key documents are identified which will enable the reader to address these issues in greater depth.

After Reading This Chapter You Will Be Able to

- *Identify the main changes in the new public health landscape.*
- *Identify the meaning of empowerment and agency in terms of public health.*
- *Recognise the role that public health professionals need to adopt to empower communities.*
- *Identify some ways in which public health can be promoted by local communities.*

M. Almond (✉)
University of East London, London E16 2RD, UK
e-mail: M.Almond@uel.ac.uk; matthewalmond@me.com

K. Regmi (ed.), *Decentralizing Health Services: A Global Perspective*,
DOI 10.1007/978-1-4614-9071-5_9,

Introduction

Over the past few years, there have been major changes in the landscape of government and as a consequence how the promotion of better health is involved. In addition the austerity measures and the severe cuts in public spending have cast a shadow on how public health programmes can be effectively delivered. This chapter will identify these changes and their implications for public health and health professionals.

The idea of empowerment has had a major impact on development work and community action but the theoretical principles underpinning this work have only just began to influence work in public health. Thus, it is important to devote time to discussing the meaning of empowerment for individuals and communities because this will have a major influence on how public health professionals put this theory into practice.

Finally, practical ways of putting theory into practice will be outlined together with suggestions for exploring the growing literature in this area.

At the end of each section, a number of questions have been posed to enable the reader to pursue new lines of inquiry and develop greater insight into the role of empowerment in public health.

The Changing Landscape

When the government launched its 5-year policy programme in 2010 (Cabinet Office 2010a), they did so in the belief that it was time for a fundamental shift of power from Westminster to people. They promoted decentralization and democratic engagement, and they ended the era of top-down government by giving new powers to local councils, communities, neighbourhoods and individuals.

The Coalition considered that governments prevent people from getting involved in their local communities and therefore they should step back and create a new driving force from the grassroots, whilst Labour saw government as providing an enabling role in supporting greater levels of participation.

Whether this vision will be translated into positive change with a real transfer of power and greater public participation to improve local communities and improve health remains a challenge to be fulfilled. The austerity measures and severe cuts in public spending introduced by the Coalition Government will have a major impact on many people and their communities but the kind of impact it will have on levels of participation and involvement remains to be seen. In April 2011, Baroness Warsi (2011), speaking on building a new culture of social responsibility, made the following points: a change is needed in society and we need a "responsibility revolution" which is about a conversion of the heart and mind, and it is a problem that together we can do something about. Responsibility is more about what an individual does and less about what the government can do. This cannot be achieved by government policy alone. It needs a smarter state and an empowered society. The change in government in 2010 has generated a different approach to community participation; the new Coalition Government's Big Society agenda (Cabinet Office 2010b; Cameron 2010) represents a significant shift in power and cultural change because it attempts to redistribute power from the Whitehall elites to local government and local communities. Ideally, the Coalition Government would like to see local communities take over the running of some public services but also playing a more active role in local planning.

Discussion Questions

How does the new Coalition Government interpret the move to transfer power to local communities?

In what ways can the idea of a Big Society be translated into practical steps that can empower health-related behaviour in local communities?

What are the differences between the previous Labour Government approach to devolving power and those of the new Coalition Government?

Public Health

The White Paper Healthy Lives, Healthy People (2011) sets out the government's new direction and future for public health. Health improvement will be directed locally with local authorities in the driving seat, supported by the latest evidence on behaviour change from a new Public Health England. To ensure public health is responsive to the different needs of each community, the government aims to create local freedom, accountability and ring-fenced health improvement budgets. It sets out how local public health leadership and responsibility will be returned to and strengthened within local government. In the new vision, each local authority and their individual Director of Public Health will act as strategic public health leaders for their local population and will deploy resources making sure that people's health and well-being is at the heart of everything local councils do.

The government's view is that society, government and individuals share collective responsibility for public health and the new public health system will encourage all to play their part in improving and protecting the nation's health and well-being. In order to promote this, a public health Responsibility Deal will be established with industry, the voluntary sector, non-governmental organisations and leading experts from the field. The intention is to make healthy lifestyles easier to achieve.

The past 2 years have seen a major reform within public health. From April 2013, local authorities have taken on board the main responsibility for coordinating local efforts to improve public health, to protect the health and well-being of the public, address health inequalities and ensure that that they can effectively put in place appropriate services to promote population health.

Health and Wellbeing Boards (HWBs) will have a statutory duty to involve local people in the preparation of a Joint Health and Wellbeing Strategy (JHWS) to meet the needs identified in the Joint Strategic Needs Assessment (JSNA). This strategy will examine the redesigning and reshaping of services and how health and social care can ensure joined-up collaboration with other associated services. The needs of the whole community and particularly those who experience inequalities and those that find it difficult to access services will have to be carefully considered and addressed. Each Joint Health and Wellbeing Strategy will be unique as they address the needs of a local area.

The role of the new Public Health England (PHE) in providing national support and co-ordination has many implications. In the spirit of localism, the government expects that PHE will have a more supportive role for local strategies and implementation. Directors of Public Health will be employed by local authorities and be responsible to them and not to Public Health England. PHE will have a commitment to supporting local action and will avoid prescriptive guidance that would be contrary to the principles of localism. At this stage it is difficult to ascertain how this relationship will work out in practice.

Discussion Questions

What are the powers of Health and Wellbeing Boards to improve public health?

What can local authorities do to engage with the public and promote better health?

What Challenges Does This Represent?

The challenge in this process will be to ascertain who the local decision makers are within the different local structures and who will work with them to develop a shared agenda of what is achievable and how everyone can collaborate and be involved. The participation of local decision makers with organisations who can contribute to health and well-being as well as members of the public in a local area represents a significant challenge. The draft guidance for Joint Health and Wellbeing Boards does not identify how JHWSs will engage with marginalised, vulnerable or excluded groups where deep inequalities are likely.

On the Health and Wellbeing Boards, there is no statutory representation for voluntary and community sectors (VCS). The Department of Health in July 2012 published draft guidance for JHWSs and JSNAs for consultation and highlighted the potential for local VCS to be represented on the HWB. They also indicated that there was scope for additional members of the HWB such as service providers, health and care professionals as well as criminal justice representatives.

The role of Healthwatch (http://www.healthwatch.co.uk) as a champion of the consumer has a statutory place on the HWB. As a result Healthwatch England will provide national leadership for local Healthwatch organisations. The government has also indicated that they will be expected to harness the expertise of the voluntary sector and others at local level.

However, these challenges only highlight the complexity of who participates in the development of a coherent public health strategy and who is responsible for its effective delivery. The background of cuts to public funding and the fundamental changes to public health promotion generates a scenario in which many service providers as well as the public will have considerable concerns about the transition to a new public health role and their ability to influence change at a local level.

Discussion Questions

What implications does a 'shared agenda' have for Health and Wellbeing Boards?

What does 'authentic public engagement' in promoting better health mean in practice?

The Meaning of 'Public' in Public Health

When one considers the meaning of the adjective 'public', we have to assume that at least some aspect of the 'public' must be involved in any discussions of public health. The meaning of 'pubic' in public health was discussed by Vertweij (2007) in his very comprehensive analysis of the concept where he provided very clear insights. Nevertheless, little attempt has been made to develop a better understanding of this term. Following Vertweij's insights, a coherent vision of the term 'public' and its relationship to the health of the public and interventions by the public might be useful in meeting the challenges of the new public health landscape.

When we speak of public health, we are not referring to the state of health of the public but to a practice or set of interventions aimed at the promotion and protection of the public, in other words, the organised and collective efforts of a community to improve health. Thus, the objectives and interventions of public health are 'public'. However, there is another important sense in which the efforts of public heath can be considered to be collective. In order to be successful, public health interventions have to involve the active commitment of members of the public. This means that many interventions need individual citizens to participate (e.g. vaccination programme, no smoking campaigns, not drinking and driving) to ensure their overall success. Also, it could mean that some public health interventions require individuals to take personal care of their own health. In the same way, participation by individuals in a public health programme (e.g. achieving high rates of vaccination) can lead to collective efforts being more effective. In this way, public health benefits are achieved through collective effort rather than individual endeavour.

Nevertheless, we can argue that members of the public have some sort of obligation to participate in public health interventions on the grounds that citizens should take actions so that others are more safe. Do citizens have an obligation to contribute to the common good? Whether there is a case to be made that we have an obligation to contribute to the common good highlights the complexity of participation of the 'public' in public health promotion.

Discussion Questions

Should people have an obligation to contribute to the common good?

Empowerment

In his article on Durable Empowerment, Drydyk (2008) succinctly outlines his interpretation of empowerment and clarifies what it means. For Drydyk, to be empowered means that a person is able to make decisions and have influence over their life choices, barriers to agency and well-being freedom. He does on to say that their capacity for such decision-making and influence will have been enhanced, if they can maintain these gains with the assets and capabilities they control (individually or collectively) and the opportunity structure in which they act. In these circumstances, it is probable that they can make these gains prevail, in the face of opposition. As a result, people are better able to shape their own lives.

Empowerment as a goal is to have control over the determinants of one's quality of life and health, and empowerment as a process is to create a professional relationship with an individual client or community setting where they take control over determining both the goals of a change process and the means adopted to bring about a desired improvement. Empowerment is a concept that has been much used and discussed for a number of years. However, it is not always explicitly clarified what its central meaning is. The present paper intends to clarify what empowerment means and relate it to the goals of health promotion. One conclusion of this discussion is that empowerment can be seen as a complex goal which includes aspects of the three central concepts welfare, health and quality of life. To the extent that the aims of empowerment are health related, it can be argued that empowerment is a legitimate goal for health promotion. But empowerment is not only a goal; it can also be described as a process or as an approach. This process involves the participants in problem formulation, decision-making and action that means the experts have to relinquish some of their control and power to the people involved.

An important goal of health promotion is to make it easier for people to make healthy choices. This is not an easy task because people may not feel that they have control over their personal circumstances or the environment in which they live.

People can be empowered to take more control over the need to change and learn to make more healthy choices. In this process health professionals can facilitate this process and enable people to move towards empowerment (Koelen and Lindström 2005).

In a key paper, Tengland (2012) compares behaviour change and empowerment in the context of the ethics of health promotion strategies. In terms of empowerment he makes the point that it has two distinct meanings; the first refers to the state of an individual or a community as a goal to be achieved and relating to the control they have in their lives (in this case health-related control) and the determinants of the quality of their lives. In the second meaning, empowerment refers to the process to attain the goals and the means of working towards empowerment, health and quality of life that is directly related to professional practice. In this way, it is a process of letting the individual or the community have as much control over the processes of change that they want (Tengland 2008). The health professional is a facilitator of change and in this role they should feel that they are also an active participant in this process by enabling an individual or community to develop their own capacities, create a vision of what is possible and put in place actions to bring them about through their partnership. In this sense the empowerment process highlights that individuals have the means (internal resources) to make changes and develop in a positive direction.

One of his interesting points is the importance of the role of the professional in promoting empowerment in the context of health promotion whose knowledge should count as an available asset. The professional within a project should have a say in the matters discussed and the decisions made. If they feel their professional responsibilities are undermined, they always have the option to refrain from continuing with the project. They should be 'experts' on how to achieve an empowering process. However, this should not be taken as a professional's right to impose their will. For the professional to have an agenda, other than facilitating increased control over the processes of change in a community or a person's health-related behaviour, would contradict the definition of empowerment as a process. It is morally problematic to attempt to make participants do what they have not consciously and deliberately freely chosen (Tengland 2008). In this situation the health professional in their role as a facilitator has to be aware that people participating in a local project are more aware of 'wider' problems in their community and have knowledge and experiences (e.g. of living conditions, environmental problems, together with perhaps a past history of poor decision-making in their locality) that often a professional lacks. A number of authors have suggested that 'real' participation of those involved in projects, i.e. when people are engaged in what is important to them, is more likely to succeed, and the effects are more likely to be sustainable (Baum 2008; Laverack 2009; Syme and Ritterman 2009).

Tengland makes a number of key points associated with empowerment. He makes the case for an association with autonomy, democratic decisions and the inequalities agenda. Since active participation requires taking or sharing responsibility for what is to be achieved, and for how it is to be achieved, this can lead to the development of various kinds of knowledge, skills and 'well-being' and increase the ability for autonomy (Laverack 2006). In the same way, groups that participate in a local project can develop their 'collective autonomy', because they are engaged in deliberating, reasoning and negotiating skills and in this process can acquire tools for making democratic decisions (Laverack 2006). He goes on to propose that empowerment strategies aimed at creating more control over health can also reduce inequalities in health. In his view community projects tend to target vulnerable or disadvantaged groups who are associated with inadequate living conditions and poorer health; therefore there is a reasonable chance that empowerment projects will reduce inequalities (Laverack 2006). Empowerment as a goal is to have control over the determinants of one's quality of life, and empowerment as a process is to create a professional relationship and partnership where the individual or community takes control over the change process, determining both the goals of this process and the means to address the problem.

This implies that people can be inspired to recognise the significance of a personal resource and its potential impact on their lives. Health professionals need to recognise that it is not enough to provide people with knowledge about improving their health and provide information about opportunities; their professional skill must go way beyond this. Their knowledge and understanding needs to be applied in such a way that professionals can apply their existing knowledge base of public health so that they can develop strategies to 'know what they can do with what they know and how they are enabled to frame possibilities beyond the conventions of the present' (Bruner 2007; p. 2).

This last point is very important because public health professionals need to help individuals to acquire the power (and have the freedom) to make choices of a certain kind (informed and rational), arrived at in a certain way (noncoercive and non-indoctrinatory), feel empowered to do so and feel that they can have some control of their own lives. For the individual, capabilities are notions of freedom, in a positive sense: what real opportunities do you have regarding the life you may lead (Clark 2005).

The health professionals' role is a complex one as they need (1) to empower individuals to make informed and noncoercive lifestyle choices and to maintain this commitment, as well as (2) to empower whole communities to address the barriers that limit and inhibit their choices and put in place opportunities that can provide them with the vision and power to make changes for their own good and improve health, and (3) to provide real opportunities (and freedom) to fulfil them. In order to achieve these roles, public health professionals will have to establish a more comprehensive and inclusive set of capabilities.

Questions

What are the main interpretations of empowerment in public health?

What is meant by 'agency', 'opportunity freedom' and 'capabilities' in empowerment theory?

Can you identify guiding principles to guide the practice of health professionals to empowering communities?

Theory into Practice

The Department for Communities and Local Government has set out in a recent report (Bringing People Together in Strong, United Communities, 2013) a number of principles that can help people to come together in strong, united communities if they are encouraged and supported to:

- Have shared aspirations, values and experiences
- Have a strong sense of mutual commitments and obligations, promoting personal and social responsibility
- Take part in local and national life and decision-making
- Fulfil their potential to get on in life
- Challenge extremism and hate crime

They believe that if it is led by the people who are most concerned, action to achieve strong communities will be more effective. At first glance, the idea of community engagement in public health appears to be a low priority because there is little evidence to support specific initiatives. The National Institute for Health and Clinical Excellent (NICE) has produced an evidence guide for Community Engagement (NICE 2008) in which they make a number of recommendations to ensure that local authorities and the NHS consult and involve local communities in decisions related to policy, service delivery, managing and governance of health promotion activities and addressing the wider determinants of health. The guidance is aimed at people involved in planning, design, funding and evaluation of national, regional and local policy initiatives; commissioners and providers in public sector organisations, the voluntary sector as well as the private sector; and members of community organisations and community representatives. Within the guidance, there are recommendations and action points for all people involved in making public health accessible to all through community engagement. In addition, there are recommendations for research organisations for further research.

The Scottish Health Council (SHC 2011) has produced a report on improving quality through patient and public participation. They explored the benefits of implementing well-designed, good quality participation and engagement in healthcare services. The paper proposes that that participation can make a positive contribution to improved effectiveness, efficiency and safety within person-centred approaches to healthcare delivery. Nevertheless, they conclude that the full benefits of participation need to be combined with NHS organisations developing a positive culture of participation.

We need to put in place procedures that will enable individuals to take responsibility for their behaviour and actions to improve their health.

Within public health teams, how a practitioner works with individuals tends to involve some behavioural change approach and there is tendency to neglect *how to engage* people, especially hard to reach groups, the lonely and the disinterested. In this context, there is a need to develop training and resources for practitioners in public health to acquire the following skills and demonstrate informed practice.

How do you *reach out* to the:

- Vulnerable
- Disadvantaged
- Hard to communicate with
- Lonely or disinterested people

How do you *connect* with them?

How do you *engage* them with something that will involve them?

How do you *draw out* their confidence and willingness to engage?

In the first place public organisations like government departments, local authorities and hospitals need to establish programmes that promote the health of their own workforce. They could establish champions to promote the idea that a healthy organisation leads to better productivity and a better return on their investment. If they could capture this learning and make it readily available, it would have major implications for all other organisations.

So, for example, there are currently accreditation awards that raise awareness of better health and they stimulate a change in practices, but they reach only a small proportion of the organisations that could be involved. The accreditation process and the provision of evidence to support their application can stimulate a significant change in attitude and practice.

Healthy Early Years Accreditation Award

- Link with health-visiting teams
- Family partnerships

Healthy Schools Accreditation Award

Healthy Workplace Accreditation Award

Housing Associations/Care Homes Accreditation Award

If local authorities could provide financial support to put in place training opportunities for mentors and volunteers to provide support for settings like workplaces, schools and organisations working with older adults, their involvement could be a focus for change. This can be illustrated with a project in early years where parents were provided with training to enable them to work in early years settings or community schemes and in return they were asked to provide between 30 and 40 h of work experience. The parents were able to gain a reference and a portfolio of experiences. The early years settings and community programmes benefited from this involvement and the parents reported positive feelings and confidence with their commitment. Such volunteer schemes can enhance the work of many different organisations.

What can a local authority or public health organisations do to enable the public to take responsibility for their health and to remove the barriers to making healthy choices? The whole process of providing information on better health for the public that is easily accessible and communicates appropriate messages to stimulate change of lifestyles/behaviour or the way that people make choices is an essential start. However, local authorities and public health organisations need to go beyond this process. Putting in place consultation processes that seek feedback on the vision and direction of health initiatives or programmes needed to ensure that a wide audience is reached and given appropriate time to respond. This needs to be followed by a clear demonstration that they are responding to feedback, listening to alternative points of view and ensuring that there is a balanced response that accommodates the diversity of views. Giving people a 'voice' that is genuinely incorporated into local decision-making enables the public to develop trust in their actions, develops commitment and instigates reciprocal respect.

The following suggestions provide a basis for change:

Short-term changes

- Provide information and advice that people can actually use and understand.
- Give local people a genuine 'voice'.
- Provide support from local authority practitioners and voluntary organisations.
- Establish partnerships and collaboratives.
- Create more better training opportunities for volunteers on evidence-improved practice.

Intermediate changes

- Build the infrastructure for joined-up action.
- Establish joined-up collaboratives.
- Genuine public representation on decision-making committees.
- Establish a resource bank for local communities.

Long-term changes

- Develop shared responsibilities.
- Put in place accountability measures for joined-up practice in public health and effective practices.

At the same time, there is a need to involve individuals and different local organisations in ways that a shared vision for promoting better health can evolve and inform practice. In this way they are building a shared responsibility and joined-up action and creating an infrastructure that enables them to work together.

Finally, the infrastructure of co-operating organisations and individuals needs to generate a process whereby they are able to capture the learning (in robust ways) from their deliberations and practice so that it can inform future decisions and actions. At the same time, there need to be put in place accountability measures that demonstrate where appropriate actions to improve health and address inequalities have been taken.

There appears to be a whole wealth of informed advice and guidance that practitioners in public health can draw upon but there is little evidence-based guidance on effective interventions that medical staff have access to. In this context, there is a need to promote ways in which practitioners can *capture the learning* from their interactions with individuals and as a member of working groups. In addition to these tools, practitioners need to be part of a culture that creates time for its staff to *capture their learning* and see it as an important dimension.

Questions

What are the main recommendations of NICE guidance for community engagement?

Identify in this document—pathways through participation—(1) what creates and sustains active citizenship and (2) the main guidance that can inform the practice of community engagement professionals and public health. It can be accessed on http://pathwaysthroughparticipation.org.uk/wp-content/uploads/2011/09/Pathways-Through-Participation-final-report_Final_20110913.pdf.

Conclusion

This chapter provides some insights into the complex field of engagement in public health and role of professionals in improving the health of local communities. The changes in government and as a result the public health landscape have brought together two powerful change mechanisms that have the potential to empower local communities to bring about change in some of the threats to the health of individuals. However, public health professions need to have a far greater understanding of what is involved in the process of community engagement and what needs to be done to bring about change. There is a great deal to learn and in times of financial hardship optimism will be required to promote more informed engagement with volunteers and the building of partnerships that share a common agenda. In this context there is a need for leadership with a clear vision of what needs to be achieved and the skills to ensure that genuine public engagement in public health becomes a reality.

The recommended readings will provide the reader with a greater understanding of these complex issues.

Recommended Readings

Deneulin, S, & McGregor, J. A. (2010). The capability approach and the politics of a social conception of wellbeing. *European Journal of Social Theory, 13*(4), 501–519.
This is a useful article that addresses the capability approach in terms of social structures and institutions that enable people to pursue individual freedoms in relation to others.

Laverack, G. (2012). *Health activism: Foundations and Strategies*. London: Sage.
A very readable textbook that provides a depth of insights into promoting health.

Institute of Health Equity. (2013, March). *Working for health equity: The role of health professionals*. Available from URL: https://www.instituteofhealthequity.org/projects/working-for-health-equity-the-role-of-health-professionals
This is essential reading on health inequalities for public health professionals.

Rowson, J., Mezey, M. K., & Dellot. B. (2012). *Beyond the big society: Psychological foundations of active citizenship*. London: RSA. http://www.thersa.org/__data/assets/pdf_file/0004/565411/NEW-NEW-COVER-Beyond-Big-Society-report-V10.pdf

An insightful analysis of the nature of social capital and the hidden wealth of public engagement.

London Civic Forum. (2012). *Take Part in London's Big Society: A review of the latest evidence, policy & provision in response to Londoners' active citizenship learning needs.* (LCF Publication No. 74). London: London Civic Forum.

As the title suggests, a detailed analysis of the learning needs for active citizenship.

Brodie, E., Hughes, T., Jochum, V., Miller, S., Ockenden, N., & Warburton, D. (2012). *Pathways through participation: What creates and sustains active citizenship?* London: NCVQ and Involve. http://pathwaysthroughparticipation.org.uk/wp-content/uploads/2011/09/Pathways-Through-Participation-final-report_Final_20110913.pdf

This is an important research report because it provides an evidence basis to inform the practice of community engagement in public health.

References

Baum, F. (2008) "Social determinants of health: The key to closing the health equity gap." http://dspace.flinders.edu.au/xmlui/handle/2328/12003.

Bruner, J. (2007). *Cultivating the Possible.* Presentation at the dedication of the Jerome Bruner Building in Oxford on 13th March 2007. http://www.education.ox.ac.uk/wordpress/wp-content/uploads/2011/03/Transcript-Cultivating-the-Possible.pdf

Cabinet Office (2010a) *The Coalition: Our programme for government HM Government.*

Cabinet Office. (2010). *Building the Big Society.* London: Cabinet Office.

Cameron, D. (2010), *Big Society Speech*, 19 July 2010. Accessed at: http://www.number10.gov.uk/news/big-society-speech

Clark, D.A. (2005) The capability approach: Its development, critiques and recent advances. GPRG-WPS-032. Global Poverty Research Group and ESRC.

Department of Health (2011) *Healthy lives, healthy people: Our strategy for public health in England.* HM Government .https://www.gov.uk/government/uploads/system/uploads/attachment_data/file/151764/dh_127424.pdf.pdf

Drydyk, J. (2008). Durable Empowerment. *Journal of Global Ethics, 4*(3), 231–245.

Koelen, M. A., & Lindström, B. (2005). Making healthy choices easy choices: The role of empowerment. *European Journal of Clinical Nutrition, 59*, S10–S16.

Laverack, G. (2006). Improving health outcomes through community empowerment: A review of the literature. *J Health Popul Nutr, 24*(1), 113–120.

Laverack, G. (2009). Public health, power and empowerment. 2nd edn. Basingstoke: Palgrave MacMillan.

NICE (2008). Community engagement to improve health. *NICE public health guidance 9.* London: National Institute for Health and Clinical Excellence.

Scottish Health Council (2011). A Scottish Health Council report on improving quality through participation: a literature review of the benefits of participation in the context of NHS Scotland's Health Quality Strategy, *Health Improvement Scotland.* http://www.scottishhealthcouncil.org/publications/research/improving_quality.aspx#.Ul1QKhYbCgE.

Syme, S. L., & Ritterman, M. L. (2009). The importance of community development for health and well-being. *Community Development Investment Review, 5*(3), 1–13.

Tengland, P.-A. (2008). Empowerment: A conceptual discussion. *Health Care Analysis, 16*(2), 77–96.

Tengland, P.-A. (2012). Behavior change or empowerment: On the ethics of health-promotion strategies. *Public Health Ethics, 5*(2), 140–153.

Verweij, M. F. (2007). The meaning of 'public' in 'public health'. In A. J. Dawson & M. F. Verweij (Eds.), *Ethics, prevention, and public health* (pp. 13–29). Oxford: Oxford University Press.

Warsi, B. (2011). *Building a new culture of social responsibility.* London: Cabinet Office. https://www.gov.uk/government/speeches/building-a-new-culture-of-social-responsibility.

Chapter 10
Public–Private Partnerships as Decentralization Strategy in Health Sector

Oliver Mudyarabikwa and Krishna Regmi

Abstract Recently, there has been considerable shift towards market mechanisms encompassing different forms of partnerships to make public services more efficient and effective. Public–private partnerships (PPPs), a form of partnership, combine government resources with the private institutions to achieve government and social goals. PPPs for health now have been considered as a process or strategy of collaborating between private sector organisations and a health programme at different levels—international, regional, national and local levels. The notion of PPPs in health is to promote collaboration in order to improve health system performance as opposed to divesting in public service provision. It is also believed that PPPs would equally bring some negative effects on public service delivery. Although approaches vary from contracting, outsourcing, privatisation and PPPs, the purpose of adopting PPPs in health systems is to prioritise competition, efficiency and effectiveness in response to globalisation, changes in technology and new approaches to managing public service delivery. Is that often the case? This chapter highlights the concepts of PPPs and their roles in health care decentralization and explores to what extent private providers working in partnership with public sector departments would bring positive effects on health service delivery, care provision and health infrastructure development.

O. Mudyarabikwa (✉)
School of Health, Sport and Bioscience, University of East London, Water Lane,
Stratford Campus, London E15 4LZ, UK
e-mail: O.Mudyarabikwa@uel.ac.uk

K. Regmi
Department of Clinical Education and Leadership, Faculty of Health & Social Sciences - Institute for Health Research, University of Bedfordshire,
Putteridge Bury Campus, Room 32, Luton LU2 8LE, UK
e-mail: krishna.regmi@beds.ac.uk

K. Regmi (ed.), *Decentralizing Health Services: A Global Perspective*,
DOI 10.1007/978-1-4614-9071-5_10, © Springer Science+Business Media New York 2014

At the End of the Chapter, You Will Be Able to

- *Define the concept of public–private partnerships and examine the roles of PPPs in health care*
- *Understand the perceived benefits, risks and the drivers/enablers of public–private partnerships in health sector of decentralising through public–private partnerships in health sector*
- *Explore and discuss the PPP experience in sub-Saharan Africa and UK health sectors*

Introduction

Since 1990, public–private partnerships (PPPs) worldwide have been recognised as a key tool of public policy (Osborne 2000). The meanings of PPPs are much contested, and people interpreted this differently in different disciplines and contexts. Skelcher (2005) views PPPs as strategy which 'combine the resources of government with those of private agents (business or not for profit bodies) in order to deliver societal goals' (p. 347).

Recently, there have been considerable discussions about the roles of PPPs in health systems across the world. WHO (2012) conceptualises PPPs as a wide variety of ventures involving a diversity of arrangements, varying with regard to participants, legal status, governance, management, policy-setting prerogatives, contributions and operational roles. In this chapter, authors will examine public–private partnerships (PPPs) as a paradigm shift for decentralization within health systems. The chapter focuses on five key issues linking between decentralization and PPP in health. Decentralization and PPP concepts are defined to show ways in which the former subsumes the latter as one of the strategies through which services within health systems are increasingly being shifted from nationalised to privatised delivery along descriptions in Fig. 10.1 (p. 3). The perceived benefits and risks of PPPs within health systems are also discussed. The chapter then presents the key factors driving PPPs within health systems. Since PPPs are increasingly being used as decentralization strategy worldwide, there is an interest to understand the important preconditions for their progress within health system, and this is presented in the fourth section of this chapter. Profiles of experience with PPPs for health delivery in low- and high-income countries are finally provided in the fifth section. The experiences are drawn from sub-Saharan countries and the UK to illustrate differences and variation in complexity of PPPs adopted across health systems.

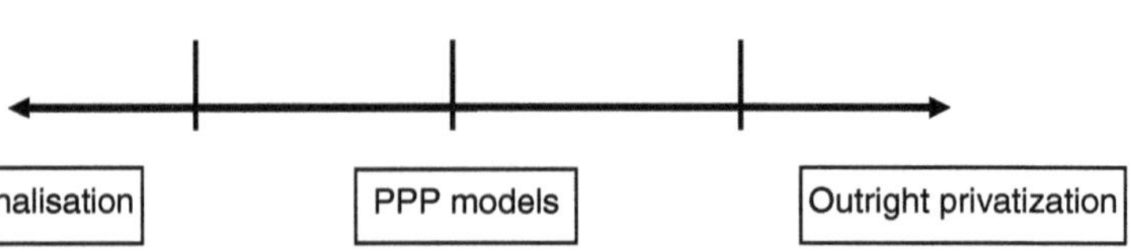

Fig. 10.1 Conceptualising PPPs and decentralization. *Source:* Adapted from Atun (2007)

Concept of Decentralization and PPPs

Decentralization is understood as the transfer of power and authority for delivery of selected functions from central to lower levels of organisations (Rondinelli 1980; Saltman et al. 2007). It does not matter whether it is a public or private organisation; decentralization technically occurs as long as power and authority for service delivery is shifted from the centre to periphery. Until the 1980s, decentralization within public organisations and health systems were perceived to involve two approaches. First, there was the transfer from national to lower governmental levels. In this case, regions or provinces or districts and local authorities were allowed enhanced power and authority to deliver functions previously provided by central government. Second, there was the transfer from national to organisational levels. In this case, hospitals or health centres and other administrative units were given enhanced power and authority over functions previously provided from national level. Thus, the essence of decentralization is that it initiates administrative rearrangements in order to transfer power and authority to deliver selected functions from the centre to peripheral levels whether within a government department or private entity.

Substantial development in public service delivery has to an extent influenced agreement to treat strategies that transfer power and responsibility to deliver health functions from public to private providers as decentralization (Atun 2007; Bennett et al. 1997). Health functions that can be potentially shifted for delivery by private providers fall under the following broad categories involving (1) service delivery, (2) care provision, (3) financing and (4) health infrastructure development. The functions can be delivered when the private providers operate individually and/or jointly in partnership with public sector departments. The scope of this chapter concerns a discussion of private providers working in partnership with public sector departments to deliver any of the functions between service delivery, care provision and health infrastructure development.

Decentralization can take place either vertically or horizontally. Mills et al. (1990) argue that within say a Ministry of Health, vertical decentralization transfers power and service delivery from the headquarters to regional or district health offices. This decentralization involves deconcentrating power, authority and responsibility for health functions from the headquarters to lower administrative governmental levels. Horizontal decentralization takes place when the ministry devolves power and authority for delivery of health services to other ministries and governmental departments (Rondinelli 1983). In Nepal, for example, the Nepalese Rural Development Foundation (2005) advocates transfer of enhanced power and responsibility for health activities to the Ministry of Local Government or local authorities. The recipients of enhanced roles should lie outside of the Ministry of Health's direct control for horizontal decentralization to take place.

Alternatively, decentralization can involve extensive delegation of power and authority to deliver health functions to semi-autonomous and private entities. Traditionally, this trend was not practised in public administration where preference was to enhance power and authority of departments that are directly controlled by the government. This has influenced disagreement on what really constitute decentralization (Savas 2000; Saltman et al. 2007). However, a number of analysts (e.g. Mills et al. 1990; Saltman 2003; Bossert 1998) argue that within health systems, activities that involve semi-autonomous and private organisations, whether working independently or in partnerships with the government, should be considered in decentralization discourse. This chapter's remit is to locate public private partnerships within decentralization discourse. The merits and demerits of involving semi-autonomous and private organisations in health service delivery are reserved for consideration in other sections of this book.

Public–private partnerships (PPPs) involve government formalising working relationships with non-governmental organisations as a way of collaborating to deliver desired public functions (World Bank 2006). PPPs for health have been considered as a process or strategy of collaborating between private sector organisations and a health programme at different levels—international, regional, national and local levels (Walley and Wright 2010). Thus, the definition adopted for this chapter is that PPPs are a form of decentralization that concerns government collaborating with the wide range of non-governmental organisations in public service delivery, which is echoed with the concept of WHO (2012). The involved non-governmental organisations may be private companies, voluntary organisations or even community groups with interests in given health functions. Such a broad definition risks disagreement with some analysts who consider efforts that promote involvement of private companies in public service delivery as privatisation (Savas 2000). But applying Saltman et al. 2007 and Atun's (2007) logic, PPPs and privatisation are distinct stages within the nationalisation–privatisation continuum that is described in Fig. 10.1.

Renda and Schrefler's (2006) argument that PPPs mainly involve transferring assets and responsibility to deliver public service from the public to private organisations also reinforces their being distinct from privatisation. An important point that is raised by World Bank (2006) is that with PPPs, the government's underlying motive is always to promote collaboration in order to improve health system performance as opposed to divesting in public service provision. Thus, PPPs essentially represent changes in ways public service is conventionally provided. It is therefore logical to recognise them as a decentralization strategy that is backed with legal or statutory arrangements unlike the conventional trends in public administration.

Perceived Benefits and Risks of Decentralising Through PPPs in Health Sector

There has been a debate flying over few decades about the role of private and public sectors. This section outlines the justifications for governments opting for PPPs as decentralization strategy in health sectors. An examination of the arguments shows that the concepts of decentralization and PPPs are linked in the sense that they share more or less similar benefits and risks. And the benefits and risks are from the standpoint of the policymakers, health professionals, analysts and consumers.

The Benefits

Using PPPs as decentralization strategy in health sectors has been recommended in many countries across the world. It is generally believed that private sector would be more 'efficient and provides higher quality services' (Walley and Wright 2010, p. 109). Even some organisations argue that 'private sector offers all the answers to public health problems in developing nations' (p. 109). Other proponents also cite a number of objectives that can be fulfilled within health sectors better than when governments act alone to deliver selected services. In particular, the objectives listed in Table 10.1 below are considered appropriate for this analysis. An important linkage between the concepts of decentralization and public–private partnerships (PPPs) relates to the strength and similarity of rationale observed to justify the strategies when used within health sector (Table 10.1).

A number of the benefits cited revolve around risk transfer from the public to the private sector partners and in some cases the sharing of risks for public service delivery between the public and private partners. For example, the World Bank (2006) and the World Health Organization (WHO) (2000) argue that PPPs may help governments to reduce administrative and financial burdens that are usually associated with public delivery of the functions. There is also the argument that despite rapid economic growth and social transformation in many developed and developing nations, countries continue to face challenges in ensuring access to quality health care services for their populations. Adopting PPPs is therefore an important innovative approach in delivering health care services (Asian Development Bank 2012). The private sector partners are presumed to have administrative skills that the public sector can exploit to improve service delivery without sidetracking public sector objectives. At the same time, the private sector partners come with financial resources that augment or replace what otherwise the public sector would be expected to provide. This helps in transferring and/or sharing risks for health service delivery.

Another benefit often cited relates to PPPs' ability to increase efficiency and effectiveness of health services (Wollmann 1990). It is argued that private sector

Table 10.1 Rationale for decentralization and PPPs within health sector

Perceived benefit to government	Decentralization	PPPs
Less administrative and financial burden	√√	√√
More efficient and effective service delivery	√√	√√
Access additional resources, skills and expertise	√√	√√
Better value for money in service delivery	√√	√√
Diversity and competition in service delivery	√√	√√
Improved technology and innovation in services	√√	√√
Responsiveness to consumer expectations	√√	√√
Democracy and voice to service purchasers and users	√√	√√
Specialisation in service delivery	√	√

√√—strong link of the benefit to strategy or (√) weak link of the benefit to strategy management systems prioritise efficiency in their activities in order to achieve value for money in service delivery. The government therefore benefits because the private sector partners use their skills and management practices to deliver more public services with as minimum resources as possible. Thus, there is higher cost-effective service delivery through both decentralization and PPPs. In fact, both the World Bank (1993) and WHO (2000) strongly argue that a great deal of public sector resources is wasted because government staff lack skills to cost-effectively deliver services. Yet working in partnership with the private sector may help to solve the problems of inefficiency and ineffective delivery of health services.

Proponents of PPPs also argue that the strategy helps the government to promote diversity within health systems (Atun 2007; Milburn 2004a, b). Whatever the PPP arrangement's purpose, there is the notion that diversity generates competition in the decentralised function. This in turn triggers reductions in cost per unit of services delivered to ultimately improve the relative efficiency health systems (Costa-Font and Rico 2006). Besides suppressing the cost of services, diversity and competition due to PPPs also increase choice for purchasers and consumers (Atun 2007). Since the 1990s, many health systems have been under pressure from especially international organisations to reform the ways health systems are managed by giving extended responsibilities to private sectors (Stingl and Wilson 1996; Mwale 1999). The World Bank (2004) particularly recommends health systems working in partnerships with private sectors in order to achieve desirable efficiency, equity and pro-poor health objectives.

One of the strengths associated with the private sector partners in health sector concerns their ability to innovate and use better technology in order to improve the quality of services along demand and expectations of consumers (Milburn 2004a, b; Normand 2012). The attraction of PPPs therefore emanates from the government pursuit for quality and keeping up to date with improvements in health care technology in order to satisfy consumer demand. According to Milburn (2004a, b), knowledgeable patients are more likely to prefer private than public sector services in search for better technology. So, PPPs may not only increase responsiveness to patients' demand for increased quality and better technology. They may also be a way of government controlling private activities and retaining influence over health activities that the private providers have to provide. There is interest on the part of government to reduce market failures within health sector. Hence, PPPs being potentially viewed as a better compromise between the two extremes of nationalisation and outright privatisation of health service delivery.

There are also implied economic and political arguments for decentralising health activities through PPPs. One of the issues that are seldom discussed concerns pressure exerted on governments to liberalise economic activities. This includes recommendations for substituting government role for multiple providers in health and other social services. Under the circumstances of resource shortage and budgetary cutbacks for public services, it is presumed that involving private providers, whether directly or in partnerships, in all economic activities helps the government to mitigate resource shortfalls (World Bank 1993; Rajasulochana and Dash 2010). Furthermore, there is the notion that the private providers that the governments are urged to engage are also citizens with legitimate rights to participate in national economic activities. The implications are that PPPs may be perceived as a strategy for opening up economies in line with philosophies of citizenship and democracy promoted by the influential international bodies. The World Health Organization (WHO) (2000) also argue that PPPs improve health system performance in the sense that the selected services will be delivered by people that are specialists in those activities rather than by health workers who may be untrained for non-health tasks. This relieves staff of daunting administrative and financial burdens, leaving them to focus on caring for patients. Hence, the argument that decentralising through PPPs may help to improve the quality of services, especially when responsibilities are allocated on the basis of suitability and ability to perform by all citizens.

The Risks

From the above discussion, it is clear that the objective of public–private partnerships (PPPs) in health sector may convey a number of benefits. These range from efficiency, quality improvement and competition-driven patient choice to innovative technology that is responsive to consumer needs and enhanced social solidarity when citizens get involved in national health activities.

However, several authors (Bossert 1998; Gaffney et al. 1999; Saltman et al. 2007; Aldred 2006; Beck et al. 2009) suggest that PPPs present a number of both opportunities and risks in decentralising health functions. The major concern is that PPPs within health sector have not been able to show convincing evidence about their ability to deliver on the anticipated benefits. Table 10.2 below shows some of the often cited risks associated with decentralization and PPPs within health sector. The table also indicates the extent to which the perceived risks aptly describe either or both decentralization and PPPs when implemented in health sector.

An important challenge in implementing decentralization and PPPs in health sector concerns issues around public sector workers' role to monitor and supervise activities of the PPPs set up to deliver the decentralised functions. Studies by Beck et al. (2009) raise concern that the government rarely train or prepare public sector

Table 10.2 Risks of decentralization and PPPs within health sector

Perceived risks to health sector	Decentralization	PPPs
Administrative and financial challenges in monitoring	√√	√√
Inadequate skills and expertise by recipients of roles	√	√√
Increased cost and neglect of decentralised services	√	√√
Lack of experience/commitment to public sector goals		√√
Reduced competition and growth of monopolies		√√
Mosaic providers and coordination challenges	√	√√
Privatisation of decentralised functions	√	√√

√√—strong link of the risk to strategy or (√) weak link of the risk to strategy workers in assuming the roles to monitor and supervise PPPs. The result is that the staff lack skills and take too long to develop effective expertise in administrative and financial matters of monitoring the partnerships. Thus, partly for this reason, some have argued that PPPs within health sector have not been able to demonstrate convincing evidence about their effectiveness within health sector (Boyle and Harrison 2000). Walley and Wright (2010, p.109) highlight that 'private sector operates as evil profiteers, contributing nothing to the public health'. In the UK, studies of the National Health Service (NHS) experience have associated PPPs with increased cost in service delivery (Gaffney et al. 1999; Pollock et al. 2005; Aldred 2006). There are strong arguments that PPPs have the risk of financing health activities through expensive borrowing from private banks. In one way or the other, private borrowing has the effect of transferring interest repayments to the public sector. At the macroeconomic level, the ripple effects include escalating health care costs that are more often than not funded by the government (Pollock et al. 2005). One of the consequences is that government investment in additional programmes that are essential from the standpoint of consumers may be curtailed. Thus, PPPs may mean that the private partners only assume superficial role to deliver and manage health service, while in reality the risk to finance is retained by the government. There is a legitimate argument that the health sector is unlike other sectors (e.g. transport, communication or manufacturing) which can adopt market mechanisms with minimum adverse effects on patient welfare. The unique nature is the reason why health sectors in many countries across the world have some form of protection against extended private participation (Equinet 2007).

But governments' efforts to protect health systems may mean that when they participate, private partners lack the benefit of prior experience in health sector issues. Consequently, PPPs risk failing to effectively deliver the decentralised functions especially by those participating in health services for the first time. Furthermore, some critics argue that the private partners either lack commitment or their interests mismatch the primary goals that government may intend to achieve through PPPs. An important problem observed by Aldred (2006) and Gaffney et al. (1999) is that profit motive of the private partners almost always tempts most PPPs to ration or neglect high cost but essential health services. Thus, PPPs risk cutting back on service availability especially where the public sector staff lack skills to monitor and power to influence compliance with the contracts by the private partners. Work by Fitzsimmons (2009) and Beck et al. (2009) actually attribute PPPs' ineffectiveness in delivering against their intentions to inadequate preparation and empowering of civil servants to monitor and supervise decentralised functions by the government.

An important reason why PPPs as decentralization strategy may be viewed unfavourably is to do with occasional market failure within health sectors. Research on effectiveness of PPPs has shown that adverse selection of patients, inefficient allocation of resources and information asymmetries influence progress against intended benefits more than the ways in which PPPs are designed (World Bank 1993; Perrot 2006; Renda and Schrefler 2006; Equinet 2007; Rajasulochana and Dash 2010). There is also cultural inertia by the private partners to shift from profit towards altruistic practices that are consistent with most health care objectives. Aldred (2006) also observes another important cultural factor that describes threats from

PPPs. While its exact mechanisms are complex, she raises the dangers of PPPs evolving into huge monolithic corporate entities that may be too big and influential for the health departments to regulate. The effects include reduced competition in service delivery and missed opportunities to benefit from diversity and wider patient choice despite them being proffered to rationalise PPPs within the health sector.

In some countries, there is concern that unless PPPs are stringently regulated, health systems may experience problems associated with fragmentation. This concern arises largely from observations that when health service providers are too mosaic, coordination of national activities is problematic and causes rapid growth in costs. Yet PPPs are viewed as a strategy to conceal government debt and costs of service delivery (Rajasulochana and Dash 2010). There is chance that inequities in health are risked especially in absence of government incentivising PPPs to invest in perceived less profitable public goods as safety nets for ordinary consumers. According to Pollock and Price (2006), PPPs also risk being used as the springboard for privatisation of health services. It does not matter whether the privatisation is intended or unintended. The paramount concern is that privatisation comes with several significant problems pointing at inequities that governments have the primary role to address.

It is clear that both decentralization and public–private partnerships (PPPs) have discrete benefits and risks, yet they are jointly adopted in many health systems. In fact, simultaneous decentralization has substantially advanced to an extent that it is no longer a case of either internal decentralization (within health departments) or using PPPs to improve health system performance. For several reasons, health systems choose to decentralise through one way or the other. Walley and Wright (2010) nicely capture the remit of PPPs in health by noting that:

> 'When we discussed financing, it becomes clear that there is a strong case for public financing of health systems—at least, a substantial minimum portion of them—to ensure social solidarity, risk-sharing and access for the poorest. When it comes to provision, however, there are less consensus on the public and private roles. Perhaps more than public or private status, what matters is the context, the incentives and the management framework which governs a facility'. (p. 109)

Activity 1

What is your understanding of PPPs? List down any three advantages and disadvantages of PPPs in health sector.

The Drivers of Public–Private Partnerships in Health Sector

To a large extent, the factors that drive public–private partners (PPPs) tend to emphasise economic, technological and societal changes on the ways public services are delivered. The factors are fuelled by changes in people's perceptions about approaches to improve the management of public services. Therefore, when viewed together, the following contextual factors are important drivers for PPPs within health sectors: (1) new approaches to public service management, (2) increased cost of health care and the need to mobilise resources for public service, (3) globalisation of economic activities including health and social care, (4) improvements in technology and managerial changes and (5) increased consumer expectations.

New Public Management

New public management (NPM) advocates private sector management techniques and market mechanisms in order to achieve success in government services. There is the underpinning perception that efficiency and effectiveness in service delivery achieved in the private sector is attributable to unique private management techniques and market mechanisms used (Pollit et al. 1998). So, when applied within health sector, NPM emphasises the shifting of health service roles (e.g. the management and operationalisation of selected health functions) from central government to peripheral units including private providers, financiers, community groups and a host of other non-governmental organisations. Although central government is expected to retain the role to regulate the decentralised functions, better health care outcomes are anticipated than would have been the case through government-led management practices. Proponents of NPM therefore argue that it makes sense for government to either privatise or work in partnerships with the private sector in order to improve health system performance (World Bank 1993; WHO 2000).

The European Observatory on Health Care Systems (2002) observes that a number of countries are increasingly substituting private provision and management practices for government role because of their perceived appropriateness within health. To a large extent, this approach to public service delivery is a worldwide phenomenon driven by the NPM ideas (Pollit et al. 1998; Saltman 2003). For example, since the 1990s, successive governments in the UK have been prioritising performance management compared to active role in administering NHS service delivery. Government bureaucracy within the NHS is replaced with regulated market mechanisms under the 'Third Way' (see Table 10.3) approach that in many ways mimic the NPM (Powell 2000).

Table 10.3 Dimensions of the 'Third Way' and connections to NPM

Delivery dimensions	Old labour	The third way	New right
Approach	Leveller	Investor	Deregulator
Outcome	Equality	Inclusion	Inequality
Mixed economy of welfare	State	Public/private civil society	Private
Mode	Command and control		Competition
Citizenship	Rights	Cooperation/partnership	Responsibility
Accountability	Central state/national	Both	Market/local
Social expenditure	High	Both?	Low
		Pragmatic	

Source: Adapted from Powell (2000), p. 42

As described in Table 10.3, NHS activities are delivered and managed through processes of contracting, public–private partnerships (PPPs), internal markets and occasional privatisation of non-clinical services (Saltman et al. 2007; McKee et al. 2006).

However, some critics are concerned about the suboptimal impact of NPM when applied in health sector. Stevens (2004) argue that private management practices fundamentally remove government role in guaranteeing equity and accountability in health. This has been supported by the work done by Pollock (2007) and Gaffney et al. (1999) who point at pro-market initiatives within the British NHS' effect of increasing health care costs. They also suggest that private management practices have failed to deliver against the anticipated efficiency and effectiveness benefits claimed by the government.

Resource Mobilisation

One important paradox in public administration is that people are unwilling to pay more taxes, yet they are not prepared to also demand less of the health services. It forces governments to explore strategies for sustaining and increasing service delivery without recourse to public funds. Thus, from government standpoint, public–private partnerships (PPPs), contracting or privatisation of selected health activities helps to (1) mobilise resources without burdening taxpayers and (2) substitute government so that better value for money is achieved with available public funds.

This is important because the cost of providing health care and services is ever escalating due to public sector staff being averse to management practices that save money in situations of declining budgets for health (World Bank 1993, 2004). The World Health Organization (WHO) (2000) also argues that there is wastage of public funds because of government's tendency to invest in less cost-effective health interventions. They therefore stress the beneficial effects of different models of PPPs and application of market mechanisms in health. According to Milburn (2004a, b), PPPs simultaneously mitigate financial shortages and mobilise equipment, technical skills and expertise abundant and otherwise suboptimally utilised in the private sector. Within developed economies—mainly the UK and central Europe—to some extent health sector reforms favouring PPPs have been influenced by governments' desire to mitigate shortage of resource needed for governments to sustain health care provision (Saltman et al. 2007). Considering the economic recession and financial liquidity problems experienced across the world between 2009 and 2012, it may be legitimate for governments to be inclined to using PPPs as alternative sources of health care finance.

Globalisation

There are also global changes that in many ways induce health systems to adopt public–private partnerships (PPPs) as decentralization strategy. Globalisation increases intensity of international competition in health. It also gives patients better patient knowledge and increased consumer demand and expectations in relation to diversity, quality, relevance and cost of services. No government wants to be found wanting in terms of delivering its health care responsibilities. These changes therefore more or less compel governments to adopt strategies that may help in meeting patient and consumer expectations more appropriately. Otherwise, there are risks of people leaving their countries to seek health care from other countries as regional and international health care boundaries are blurred by globalisation.

The risks are usually averted through restructuring of the ways public service is delivered within countries. For example, protected health systems in the former communist countries were restructured to accept public–private mix provision. Where open economies already existed, health care and services as well as education previously delivered through government monopoly are decentralised to public–private partnerships or delivered through privatisation, contracting and other market-based initiatives. Furthermore, international development agencies like the World Bank, International Monetary Fund and the WHO encourage these as strategies for improving health system performance in the wake of overall decline of budgets for public service.

Technology and Managerial Changes

Technological changes and managerial practices are also the pillars of public–private partnerships (PPPs) in health. Health care technology should not be considered only in terms of new techniques, equipment or drugs. It also concerns better understanding as well as changes in ideas to reduce cost of health outputs and outcomes. This broader definition is appropriate to understand the drivers for PPPs in health (Normand 2012). PPPs are generally perceived as more responsive to changes in technology compared to government management practices. There is government recognition of the importance of investing in processes that keep pace with improvements in technology in order to reduce costs and meet consumer demand for services that reflect improvements in technology. Strategies that encourage private sector involvement are therefore viewed to have the benefits of speed and appropriate response to consumer demands and expectations.

Managerial changes are important in the sense that current focus of most governments is on improving the inputs and processes that are central to production of essential health care and service outcomes. In general, the private sector is perceived to have better skills, expertise and resourcefulness than the government in executing the managerial changes. Strategies like PPPs are therefore perceived to improve resource allocation and utilisation and organisational rearrangements while retaining government influence. This makes the health systems competitive and enhances performance and the quality of services.

Increased Consumer Expectations

There is a linear relationship between globalisation and changes in technology on one hand and rising consumer demands and expectations in health. Works by Atun (2007) and Normand (2012) indicate that both globalisation and technology create patients' awareness about alternatives in health care interventions. The end result is that patients increasingly demand choice and better access because they are more knowledgeable about innovations that improve quality of life. They expect health systems to meet their needs and conform to international standards without making them bear the burden of higher cost. For example, in the UK, NHS patients are believed to be intolerant to drab services provided at public facilities (Milburn 2004a, b). So PPPs are justified on the grounds of helping the government to meet patient expectations in order to curtail their drift to unaffordable private sectors. There is also the perception that unmet consumer expectations go against the founding ethos of the NHS and can therefore politically risky for the government (Milburn 2004a, b).

Preconditions for Progress with PPPs

One key challenge to progress with PPPs is the level of scrutiny provided by the public. Most critics, purchasers and service users perceive PPPs as politically conceived to cover for government cuts on investment in health. It implies that the public may be unaware or do not understand PPP benefits and how they may help the health sector to mobilise local resources in order to improve outputs and care and service outcomes. So, the general call may be for proponents to revisit rationale for PPPs in order to mesh them with the public's real expectations from decentralising health activities.

In addition, and depending on the nature of health functions targeted for decentralization, institutional capacity development may be required (McKee et al. 2006). The majority of PPPs in health are monitored by health workers who may be found wanting for experience in monitoring administrative and financial aspects of PPPs (World Bank 2006). Research in the English NHS has shown that strong institutional capacity in planning and developing PPPs is crucial for local staff to avoid relying on external technical assistance (King's Fund 2008).

Another important precondition is the legal frameworks to give PPPs the necessary security of status especially since they use public assets and resources along more or less private interests (Bennett et al. 1997). PPP laws are designed to resolve specific and potential problems known to occur as a result of operationalising the partnership. Per se, legal frameworks cannot impede progress with PPPs unless expectations and deliverables by the partners and PPP mechanisms are unclear. The legal frameworks are also linked to the regulatory frameworks. In this case, public sector staff and stakeholders entrusted with monitoring PPP activities perform better if they are conversant with the contexts and procedures for executing effective PPPs.

A seldom mentioned precondition for successful PPPs regards private providers' readiness to assume responsibility over functions they may lack familiarity with. When comparing between developed and low-income countries, differences in impact give the impression that existence of well-developed and experienced private sectors is important precondition for successful PPPs. In general, where the private sector is well developed, PPP impact is very high. And the converse is also true.

PPP Experience in Sub-Saharan Africa and UK Health Sectors

Different PPP models have substantially helped to improve performance of health systems in high- and low-income countries. However, noticeable differences exist in terms of ingenuity at initiating and managing new models to enhance their ability to deliver the anticipated benefits considering the complex nature of health care environments. Unless initiated and adopted with foreign technical assistance, health systems in low-income countries are prone to adopting simple and time-tested PPP models. Those in high-income countries tend to explore opportunities for innovation in order to try new models for a variety of health care activities. For example, in low-income countries, only care and services are delivered through PPPs that contract and outsource from individual and private providers (Bennett et al. 1997). They may also devolve service delivery to local authorities or municipalities (Bennett 1990). But in high-income countries, it is now common for public sector health care physical infrastructure to be delivered and managed through PPP arrangements and resources (McKee et al. 2006). Such initiative is missing in developing countries despite the lack of government funding for public sector hospitals and health centres.

PPPs in Sub-Saharan Africa

Since the colonial years, African countries have accessed private sector resources to fund health care (Mills et al. 1990). The objective was to facilitate private for-profit providers serving consumption for the affluent urban populations. In remote and rural areas inaccessible to government structures, the private not-for-profit providers would service the indigent population. According to Bennett et al. (1997), a considerable proportion of consumers in sub-Saharan Africa received health care from the private not-for-profit providers. Work by the Regional Network for Equity in Health in Eastern and Southern Africa (Equinet) (2007) indicates that health care partnerships are predominant in Southern, Eastern, Central and Western Africa. In these regions, missionaries (faith-based providers) work in partnership with central governments to contribute up to 10 % of health care finance (WHO 2000) needed to provide both curative and preventive services to as much as 70 % of the rural population (Equinet 2007).

Following independence, health systems in sub-Saharan countries delegated extended roles as recognition of the importance of not-for-profit providers in improving performance. For example, in Zimbabwe, Zambia and Tanzania, the governments designate Mission Hospitals to provide district or provincial level hospital care where government facilities are inadequate (Mudyarabikwa and Madhina 2000). Such partnership arrangements are fashionable across a number of sub-Saharan countries where local private facilities may be bigger or provide wider range of services than public facilities. McPake and Hongoro (1995) observe that mining and agricultural corporations owning health facilities are occasionally contracted by government to provide clinical and preventive services to local public patients. The private health facilities are primarily for attracting or retaining employment of critical staff in remote areas. This is predominant in sub-Saharan regions where PPPs are relied upon for primary care level consumptions. However, PPPs are not often used to deliver health care physical infrastructure despite their potential as a means of funding public sector capital projects.

Experience in the UK

Public–private partnerships (PPPs) have been invariably used to decentralise health care and service delivery in several countries across Europe to the extent of making it difficult to distinguish between public and private health sectors (Saltman 2003). But the UK has been arguably at the forefront in terms of exploring opportunities to extend PPPs into other health functions. Successive UK governments have adapted PPP models traditionally reserved for decentralising infrastructure development for application within the health sector (Boyle and Harrison 2000; McKee et al. 2006). Although their level of success is variable, two prominent PPP initiatives originating from the UK concern the Private Finance Initiative (PFI) and Local Improvement Finance Trust (LIFT) designed to improve the delivery and management of hospitals and primary care buildings, respectively.

The Private Finance Initiative

The Private Finance Initiative (PFI) in health sector was a strategy introduced in 1992 to decentralise the financing, development and management of hospitals within the NHS. PFI involved central government, encouraging and supporting private companies to create consortiums that would be contracted by NHS trusts to construct desired capital assets and provide necessary operational services for periods up to 30 years. What distinguishes PFI from other PPP arrangements in health sector is that the new consortiums do not provide direct care or services to patients. Instead, their remit is to manage and maintain the new facilities for continuous availability to hospital trusts that retain the role to provide patient care and services.

Like other decentralization strategies, PFI within the health sector is criticised for a number of reasons. Several evaluations of PFI projects within the NHS (e.g. Gaffney et al. 1999, Pollock et al. 1999; Boyle and Harrison 2000; McKee et al. 2006) argue that it has pitfalls including the following risks: (1) substandard buildings due to poor workmanship, (2) poor maintenance of facilities caused by lack of health sector experience, (3) increased cost for the public sector due to expensive borrowing by the SPVs and (4) risk of rationing of essential care and services when hospital trusts strive to save in order to repay mortgages. Notwithstanding the concerns, PFI was adopted as decentralization strategy for developing health sector capital projects in several countries within the European Commission (Barretta and Ruggiero 2008).

Local Improvement Finance Trust

In many ways, Local Improvement Finance Trust (LIFT) is considered a second-generation PFI mechanism to finance primary care buildings at local levels. Typical LIFT partnership within the NHS involves the Department of Health, local Primary Care Trust (PCT) and interested private sector companies forming a partnership company—Local Improvement Finance Trust Company (LIFTCo)—to spearhead the planning, designing, construction and maintenance of desired primary care buildings. The Liftco is obligated to lease the delivered facilities to the PCT in return for agreed rentals from the latter for periods lasting to 25 years. What it means is that LIFT facilitates PCT investment in public buildings without direct recourse to government funds. It is argued that to LIFT partnerships have been key in influencing delivery of better looking, fit-for-purpose and appropriately maintained primary care buildings (King's Fund 2008; Beck et al. 2009).

Yet some critics have also raised problems of LIFT replicating the risks associated with PFI. Aldred (2006), Fitzsimmons et al. (2009), Pollock and Price (2006) and Beck et al. (2009) have used different perspectives to examine LIFT's impact on NHS primary care. Their conclusions of variable evidence for effectiveness against the intended benefits suggest that lessons learnt from PFI may have not been helpful in shaping the implementation processes. It is argued that LIFT inadvertently increases the cost of procuring primary care buildings, which triggers cutbacks in essential service delivery because PCTs hard pressed to save money in order to pay rent. A recent evaluation of LIFT (Mudyarabikwa 2012) also raised the concern about commercial secrecy in implementing LIFT. Staff at the front line feels excluded in making critical decisions about how the programme is implemented. As a result, the overall perception is that, in terms of quality, the services that LIFT offers are not commensurate to the costs and risks. Even senior managers within PCTs signed up for LIFT worry about the strategy's ability to sustain investment in public buildings given liquidity problems faced by the banks financing the partnerships. Currently, the UK government promotes 'localism' in public service procurement. In a way this may be viewed to courting to work in partnerships with individuals, community voluntary groups, charities and a raft of other public but not state-run organisations in order to deliver important social and public goals.

Activity 2: What are the ethical and operational/process-related challenges involved in PPPs in health sector? List down any five key challenges.

Conclusion

There is considerable shift towards market mechanisms encompassing different forms of PPPs to provide health care in many systems across the world. In high-income countries, health care provision has evolved substantially to being not an 'either-or' case between public and private sector involvement. Although the roles of private sectors differ significantly on the aspects of policymaking, financing, provision of services and regulation (Merson et al. 2012) and approaches vary from contracting, outsourcing, privatisation and public–private partnerships, it is evident that most health systems are now characterised by collaborative coexistence between public and private providers (Saltman et al. 2007). This is because PPPs are perceived to enhance health systems' response to consumer needs and demand for quality services (Bossert 1998; Milburn 2004a, b). Health systems that adopt PPPs are perceived to prioritise competition, efficiency and effectiveness in response to globalisation, changes in technology and new approaches to managing public service delivery (Powell 2000, Atun 2007; Normand 2012). In addition, PPPs may be a means to optimising technical skills, expertise and excess resources from the private sector to benefit service users (McKee et al. 2006; Beck et al. 2009). However, there is no consensus about the theory, conceptual process and impact of PPPs experienced within health sector. They are perceived to promote entrepreneurialism leading to assortments of inequitable outcomes in health (Aldred 2006; Gaffney et al. 1999). Furthermore, PPPs risk being stepping stone to privatisation well as expensive for the government because they are financed through private borrowing (Pollock and Price 2006). Because the private sector initiates and manages the borrowing even though government is involved in interest repayment, PPPs are viewed as a strategy to conceal public debt (Rajasulochana and Dash 2010).

Notwithstanding the lack of agreement on impact or conceptual approaches for increasing effectiveness, there is evidence for increased reliance on PPPs to deliver health functions (WHO 2000; World Bank 2006). In European high-income countries, more physical infrastructure for health is developed through PPPs than the governments (Perrot 2006; McKee et al. 2006; Saltman and Bankauskaite 2006).

So rather than wishing PPPs away, they may be taken advantage of provided governments consider to:

- Disseminate experiential information for managers, service users and stakeholders to be convinced about the impact of PPPs on health sector performance.
- Capacitate public sector staff so that they are more effective at monitoring performance of PPPs to reduce risks for questionable outcomes.
- Reduce negative perceptions by putting in place transparent procedural and regulatory frameworks so that PPPs' underlying intentions are not questioned.

There is a general observation that people are more amenable to PPP arrangements involving not-for-profit than for-profit providers. Besides covering large population groups, private not-for-profit providers are thought to prioritise equity and service-user satisfaction in health care compared to the latter whose profit motive may be disincentive to invest in less profitable services demanded by consumers.

Further Discussion

- What is needed for successful public–private partnerships in the health sector? Discuss.
- Why do you think that health care should not be left to the private market? Or should it? Discuss.
- What would be the role of private sector (contractors or consultants) in delivering effective technical assistance in both health policy development and health service delivery? Discuss.

Further Reading

Nikolic, I. A., & Maikisch, H. (2006). *Public-private partnerships and collaboration in the health sector: An overview with case studies from recent european experience*. Washington, DC: The International Bank for Reconstruction and Development/The World Bank.
This provides an overview of the topic of public–private partnerships in the health sector. This also highlights the types of PPPs and the associated benefits and risks and good practices for ensuring success.

Merson, M., Black, R., & Mills, A. (2012). *Global health: Diseases, programs, systems, and policies*. London: Jones & Bartlett Learning.
This book is a highly sensitive, multidisciplinary approach to the health challenges and offers many new and emerging perspectives, and it makes an important contribution to the field of health sciences globally.

Nishtar, S. (2004). Public—private 'partnerships' in health—a global call to action. *Health Research Policy and Systems, 2*, 5. doi:10.1186/1478-4505-2-5
This article conceptualises the meaning of public–private 'partnerships' in health sector exampling from the perspective of global context. This also highlights that the dynamics of public–private partnership arrangements might help to initiate global and country-specific actions.

References

Aldred, R. (2006). In the interests of profit, at the expense of patients: An examination of the NHS Local Improvement Finance Trust (LIFT) model: Analysing six key disadvantages. *PFI Reports for* Unison: pp. 1–21

Asian Development Bank. (2012). *Public-private partnerships in health.* Manila, Philippines: ADB Headquarters.

Atun, R. (2007). Privatisation as decentralization strategy. In R. B. Saltman, V. Bankauskaite, & K. Vrangbaek (Eds.), *Decentralization in healthcare. European Observatory on Health Systems and Policies Series* (pp. 247–266). Maidenhead: McGraw Hill/Open University Press.

Barretta, A., & Ruggiero, P. (2008). Ex-ante evaluation of PFIs within the Italian health-care sector: What is the basis for this PPP? *Health Policy Journal, 88*, 15–24.

Beck, M., Toms, S., Mannion, R., Brown, S., Fitzsimmons, D., Lunt, N., & Green, I. (2009). *The role and effectiveness of public-private partnerships (NHS LIFT) in the development of enhanced primary care premises and services.* The University of York: Report for the National Institute for Health Research Services Delivery and Organisation Programme.

Bennett, R. (1990). *Decentralisation, local governments and markets: Towards post-welfare agenda.* Oxford: Clarendon.

Bennett, S., McPake, B., & Mill, A. (1997). *Private health providers in developing countries: Serving the public interest?* London: Zed Books Ltd.

Bossert, T. (1998). Analysing the decentralization of health systems in developing countries: Decision-space, innovation and performance. *Social Science and Medicine, 47*(10), 1513–1527.

Boyle, S., & Harrison, A. (2000). *Investing in health buildings: Public-private partnerships.* London: The King's Fund.

Costa-Font, J., & Rico, A. (2006). Vertical competition in the Spanish National Health System. *Public Choice, 128*, 477–498.

Equity in Health in East and Southern Africa. (2007). *Reclaiming the resources for health: A regional analysis of equity in health in East and Southern Africa.* Zimbabwe, Harare: Weaver.

Fitzsimmons, D., Brown, S., & Beck, M. (2009). Does the UK Local Improvement Finance Trust (LIFT) Initiative improve risk management in public-private procurement? *Journal of Risk and Governance, 1*(2), 137–156.

Gaffney, D., Pollock, A. M., Price, D., & Shaoul, J. (1999). The private finance initiative: NHS Capital expenditure and the private finance initiative: Expansion or contraction? *British Medical Journal, 319*, 48–51.

King's Fund. (2008). *Under one roof: Will polyclinics deliver integrated care?* London: King's Fund.

McKee, M., Edwards, N., & Atun, R. (2006). Public private partnerships for hospitals. *Bulletin of the World Health Organisation, 84*(11), 890–896.

McPake, B., & Hongoro, C. (1995). Contracting out clinical services in Zimbabwe. *Social Science & Medicine, 41*(1), 13–24.

Merson, M., Black, R., & Mills, A. (2012). Global health: Diseases, programs, systems, and policies. London: Jones & Bartlett Learning.

Milburn, A. (2004a). *Localism: The need for a new settlement.* Speech at Demos Seminar

Milburn, A. (2004b). *The future of public-private partnerships.* Speech to the Public Private Partnership (PPP) Forum Conference. Birmingham.

Mills, A., Vaughan, J. P., et al. (1990). *Health systems decentralisation: Concepts, issues and country experiences.* Geneva, Switzerland: World Health Organisation.

Mudyarabikwa, O. (2012). Evaluation of the Planning and Implementation of Local Improvement Finance Trust (LIFT) schemes in East London. *PhD Thesis. University of East London.* London.

Mudyarabikwa, O. & Madhina, D. (2000). An assessment of incentive setting for the participation of private for-profit health care providers in Zimbabwe. *PHR-Plus: Small Applied Research No. 15.* Bethesda, USA

Mwale, G. (1999). Health reform in Zambia. *International Nursing Review, 46*, 156–157.

Normand, C. (2012). The healthcare system in Ireland: Controlling growth in expenditure and making best use of resources. In: Callan, T. (ed), *Budget Perspectives 2012* (57–74). Dublin: Economic & Social Research Institute (ESRI) Research Series 22.

Osborne, S. P. (2000). *Public-private partnerships: Theory and practice in international perspective*. London: Routledge.

Perrot, J. (2006). Different approaches to contracting in health systems. *Bulletin of the World Health Organisation, 84*(11), 859–66.

Pollit, C., Birchall, J., & Putman, K. (1998). *Decentralizing public service management*. London: Macmillan.

Pollock, A. M., Dunnigan, M. G., Gaffney, D., Price, D., & Shaoul, J. (1999). The Private Finance Initiative: Planning the "New" NHS: Downsizing for the 21st Century. *BMJ 319*, 179–84.

Pollock, A. M. (2007). PPPs and the Private Finance Initiative. Letter: *Bulletin of World Health Organisation* 85(11). Available at: www.ncbi.nlm.nih.gov/pmc/articles/PMC2636251/pdf/07-042218.pdf. (Accessed 15/06/ 2010).

Pollock, A. M. & Price, D. (2006). Privatising primary care. *British Medical Journal [Editorial]*. Aug. 2006, 565–566

Pollock, A. M., Price, D., & Player, S. (2005). *The private finance initiative: a policy built on sand. an examination of the treasury's evidence base for cost and time overrun data in value-for-money policy appraisal*. Report for Unison.

Powell, M. (2000). New Labour and The Third Way in the British Welfare State: A New and Distinctive Approach? *Critical Social Policy, 20*(1): 39–60.

Rajasulochana, S. & Dash, U. (2010). *The economics behind public-private partnerships in health sector*. Available at: http://www.cehat.org/g/uploads/PPP/rajasulochanapaper.pdf. (Accessed 15 Dec. 2011).

Renda, A. & Schrefler, L. (2006). *Public-private partnerships models and trends in the european union. director general internal policies of the union*. Brussels: Directorate A - Economic and Scientific Policy

Rondinelli, D. A. (1980). Government decentralization in comparative perspective: Theory and Practice in Developing Countries. *International Review of Administrative Sciences June 1980, 47,* 133–145.

Rural Development Foundation (RDF). (2005). *Sector devolution strategy*. Nepal: Nepal Rural Development Foundation.

Saltman, R. B. (2003). Melting public-private boundaries in European health systems. *European Journal of Public Health, 13*, 24–29.

Saltman, R. B., & Bankauskaite, V. (2006). Conceptualizing decentralization in European Health Systems: A functional perspective. *Health Economics, Policy and Law, 1*(2), 127–147.

Saltman, R. B., Bankauskaite, V., & Vrangbaek, K. (2007). *Decentralization in Healthcare. European Observatory on Health Systems and Policies Series*. Maidenhead: McGraw Hill/ Open University Press.

Savas, E. S. (2000). *Privatisation and public-private partnerships*. New York: CQ Press.

Skelcher, C. (2005). Public–private partnerships and hybridity. In E. Ferlie, L. E. Lynn, & C. Pollitt (Eds.), *Oxford handbook of public Management* (pp. 347–370). Oxford: Oxford University Press.

Stevens, S. (2004). Reform strategies for the English NHS: Incentives and local accountabilities are again likely to be emphasized in England's National Health Service. *Health Affairs, 23*(3), 37–44.

Stingl, M., & Wilson, D. M. (1996). *Efficiency versus equality: Health reform in Canada*. Canada: Fernwood Publishing.

The World Bank. (1993). *World development report 1993: Investing in health*. New York: The World Bank, Oxford University Press.

The World Bank. (2004). *World development report 2004: Making services work for poor people*. New York

The World Bank. (2006). *Public-private partnership units: What are they, and what do they do?* The World Bank Group: Financial and Private Sector Development. Vice Presidency Note Number 311.

The World Health Organisation. (2000). *The world health report 2000: Health systems improving performance*. Geneva, Switzerland: WHO.

The World Health Organisation. (2012). *Public-private partnerships for health*. Available at: http://www.who.int/trade/glossary/story077/en/ (Accessed on 23/12/12).

Walley, J., & Wright, J. (2010). *Public health: An action guide to improving health*. Oxford: Oxford University Press.

Wollmann, H. (1990). Decentralisation: What it is and why we should care. In R. Bennett (Ed.), *Decentralisation, local governments and markets: Towards post-welfare agenda*. Oxford: Clarendon.

Chapter 11
Gender Analysis and Use of Intersectionality in Health

Ritu Mahendru

Introduction

In this chapter, gender analysis is conducted from an intersectional lens to see how well the concept of gender is included at policy and research levels. Using international evidence to contextualise gender in relation to different regional experiences from the low-, middle- and high-income countries, the review demonstrates that there is poor quality information and lack of robust data that presents limitations and difficulties in terms of understanding gender inequalities in health. The chapter argues that women and men cannot be uniformly considered disadvantaged in terms of health. Inequalities are not concentrated in one gender or the other rather disadvantaged social positions that are multidimensional and are fundamental causes of gender inequities in health. Therefore, the focus needs to be on understanding health inequities rather than health inequalities, which should be explored through the intersecting domains of inclusion, exclusion and identity that have potential to explain where inequalities exist and why. The chapter argues that serious gender analysis requires an intersectional approach with a spatial dimension. Finally, it discusses how well gender in decentralised system is included at research and governance levels. It then concludes that the concepts of decentralization and health equity require women empowerment as well empowerment and involvement of those who are socially excluded at institutional levels.

R. Mahendru (✉)
42 Bayston Road, London, UK
e-mail: mahendru.ritu@gmail.com

K. Regmi (ed.), *Decentralizing Health Services: A Global Perspective*,
DOI 10.1007/978-1-4614-9071-5_11,

After Reading This Chapter You Will Be Able to

- *Conceptualise gender in health from a sociological perspective*
- *Understand gender health inequalities through social exclusion and identity frameworks*
- *Identify different social aspects that interact and intersect with gender*
- *Understand the importance of intersectionality theory for serious gender analysis*
- *Understand the relationship between gender and decentralization*

Conceptualising Gender in Health

Conceptualising gender is an overarching theoretical process, which includes understanding the changing meanings of the term itself and how it operates in everyday world. Thc concept of gender has been explored by many health professionals and academics (Connell 2012; Annandale and Hunt 2000). While sex is associated with the female and male anatomy, gender refers to the social construction of roles and identity associated with women and men. This can be understood through the notions of performativity whereby gender social roles are seen as interplay of performance that women and men carry out in accordance with their socially constructed identities. However, the ways in which people act and behave are spatially bound. In this context, the theory of 'gender performance' shifts based on spaces people occupy.

In general, there is some evidence that suggest the ways in which gender affects the health status of women and men, which is significantly influenced by their lifestyles and socially constructed roles. The roles are classified by certain socially defined feminine and masculine traits and behaviours, whereby a woman is expected to be passive, subservient and conformist and a man active and risk taker (Holland et al. 1998). These are stereotypes; stereotypes influenced by social practices lead to imbalance in health services and are often signifiers of gender inequalities in health. This is where distribution of health becomes a critical concern making gender central to the understanding of health inequalities. However, the complexities with which the concept of gender acts, interacts and impacts the delivery of health services have not been explored too well in health sciences. Health researchers have often relied on the essentialised gender categories of women and men to understand their association with specific health illnesses and conditions.

The dangers of gender stereotyping in health have been highlighted by Kuhlmann and Annandale (2010). They argue that not only evidence on gender inequalities in health is 'scattered and fragmentary', but they also argue that women and men are being excluded from health care services due to gender biases and stereotypical presumptions leading to problems of access and lack of health services in certain health areas. They assert that women's needs have been marginalised in the coronary health and gender bias is often noticed in psychotropic services due to stereotypes of women being the mentally weaker sex, and likewise a lack of mental health services for men is also noticed.

Another example of stereotypical images is that there is often an underlying assumption of men drinking and smoking more compared to women. The norms of masculine behaviour often relate to increase in alcohol consumption, binge drinking, drug use and its consequences (Obot and Room 2005). Their higher rates of cigarette smoking, gun use, employment in hazardous occupations and risk taking in recreation and driving are considered to be responsible for higher death rates. While it is true that men's risky behaviours are major contributors to negative health outcomes and causes of death, several studies now indicate that gender gaps in the prevalence of heavy episodic drinking have become small or nonexistent in some European countries (such as Ireland, Norway and the United Kingdom) but also in some developing countries such as Nigeria and Mexico (WHO 2004). It is important to draw an example of and discuss substance use and gender factors associated with drinking here, as drinking is considered to be a male practice, which has led health professionals to continue gender stereotypical practices that are potentially detrimental to the health and social positioning of women and neglect to gender-specific health services.

As we try to strike the balance between women and men and women's status catches up with men, women now have access to spaces and opportunities that they did not have before. In certain settings women are now taking as many risks as men do. Women are drinking and smoking more and experiencing more job-related stress (Yin 2007; Kolip 2010). The changing gendered and social health patterns have also been reflected in a report by the WHO (2008a) on cardiovascular diseases (CVDs). It is reported that in 2004, 60 % of deaths globally are due to non-communicable diseases and CVDs are the leading causes of death and disability in the world. The data shows that CVDs are the leading causes for almost 27 % of all deaths in men and 32 % in women, which has traditionally been assumed to be a male-specific problem.

It is estimated that 17.3 million people died from CVDs in 2008—more women die than men from CVDs. Similarly, Peden et al. (2004) in a WHO report informed that one in eight men and one in fourteen women die of injury-related diseases in the world. The organisation estimates that road traffic injuries lead to 1.2 million deaths annually and an additional 20–50 million fatal injuries, the majority of which occur in low- and middle-income countries. However, when other social development indicators are compared with injury-related illnesses such as economy and geography, one will notice that 'road traffic injuries are the leading cause of death among adolescent girls in high- and middle-income countries' (WHO 2009a, b). While this is true amongst more privileged socio-economic groups where female adolescents are engaged in risk-taking behaviours, similar patterns can be observed in women and men at the lowest socio-economic spectrum.

Gender roles are now shifting and changing in low-income countries. For instance, mining is traditionally considered a man's job and often associated with masculinity. Yet little is known about women's engagement in the mining industry from health perspectives and its forms of hazardous risks on them as well as its links to other social development and health indicators such as class, caste and geography. Please see Case Study 1.

Case Study 1

In the rural part of Rajasthan, both women and men are involved in extraction of sandstone in unsafe conditions from sedimentary rock quarries. Both female and male 'Dalit' miners work tirelessly in scorching heat in deep open pits where the air is thick with silica sand dust as a result of dry drilling of the mines using hand chisels and hammers. The health diseases women face working in hazardous conditions alongside men are tuberculosis, anaemia and chronic weakness. A study conducted by GRAVIS (2010) reports that 95 % of women miners in Jodhpur and 84, 81 and 70 % in Barmer, Makrana and Bikaner cities of Rajasthan, India, respectively, face these health problems. Occupational hazards such as neck and back problems and swollen feet due to wounds from spikes and stones in the mines are also common. While women and men face equal health risks and challenges in the mines, women remain disadvantaged. Men in these spaces are active agents in constructing and reconstructing dominant forms of masculinity, whereas women's sense of existence or belonging to the mines only comes from their husbands. What is unknown is women's extensive involvement in mining work and their involvement in hard labour from a very young age working beyond gender stereotypes.

GRAVIS reports that women are more likely to be subjected to sexual abuse in a situation where there are no or a lack of toilet facilities around mines. Additionally, the female mine workers also contribute significantly to the domestic work from fetching water to nursing ill family members and ignoring their own nutritious needs either for a male member of the family or children, making them more susceptible to other chronic diseases and illnesses. Furthermore, a majority if not all of the women working in the mines are married and work alongside their husbands. Their health status is also determined by their reproductive health. GRAVIS informed that 33 % of the female respondents in a study in Rajasthan reported working in mines during their pregnancy. Moreover, close to 41 % of the female respondents have worked in the mines until the third trimester. None of the women miners reported receiving equitable treatment or benefits during pregnancy or maternity from the mine owners.

(GRAVIS 2010).

Stereotypical images about gender roles further exacerbate health inequities making the difference between women and men more unequal and gap wider. It is true that the social construction of masculinity affects men as well as women. Men are more likely to be in dangerous jobs, and they also face problems that are gender based and gender related. While all of this is true, it can be said that men may be damaged by the social construction of masculinities; they are rarely harmed in any direct way by gender inequalities themselves (Payne and Doyal 2010).

It is important that as health professionals, we understand the biological and social similarities and differences that exist between the two genders, which refers to women and men. Biological as well as social differences and inequities make it difficult for women to achieve equality.

Difference Between Gender Equity and Equality

Before discussing gender inequalities any further, it is important to understand the difference between gender equity and equality. There are a broad range of thoughts that exist in defining what really equity and equality is and the relationship and differences between the two. However, often the terms equity and equality are used interchangeably in theory as well in practice without really finding the need to explain it. Payne and Doyal (2010) provide a detailed account of what the two terms mean and how the international policy actors perceive the two terms. They inform that we are yet to gain consensus over categorising and distinguishing terms equity at policy and programmes levels. While equality is a widely used and accepted term, equity is still gaining consensus at national and international levels. Equality is concerned with the equal social status of both women and men, whereas equity focuses on social disparities and biological differences that give rise to inequalities. Equity is a process, while equality is an eventual outcome. Equality can only be achieved by closing the gender and other social gaps, which is equity.

WHO Definitions of Equity

'an ethical concept that eludes precise definition. Synonyms are social justice and fairness, which again, could be taken to mean differently by people at different times. Equity usually deals with a predetermined standard or norm, which is considered "just" or "fair"'.

'Equity in health mainly focuses on the health of the vulnerable population in absolute rather than relative terms. A policy or programme aimed at improving the health of the most vulnerable would be seen as being equitable'.

(WHO 2008b)

Gender Gaps in Life Expectancy: Inequalities in Health?

Another debate is the one around gender gaps in life expectancy, which has led us to posit a complex explanation as to why more women die older and more men die younger? It is one of the indicators that are used to measure the health differences between women and men.

Table 11.1 Life expectancy at birth by country (World Bank 2011)

Country	Female	Male
Afghanistan	61	59
Australia	84	80
India	67	64
Lesotho	47	49
Nepal	70	68
Mali	52	50
Russia	75	63
United Kingdom	82	79
United States	81	76

It is now clear that women and men have similar cause-of-death patterns, yet they have distinctive patterns of mortality whereby women tend to live longer than men in many parts of the world. While there is no definitive answer available, the current evidence leads to biological (Yin 2007) as well social (Payne and Doyal 2010) explanations. Gender gaps and differences in mortality and life expectancy vary by country (Yin 2007), and this is true amongst groups who enjoy higher social and economic status.

In the developed part of the world, both women and men tend to enjoy higher life expectancy than those in developing world, fragile and conflict settings as shown in Table 11.1. While there is not much female and male disadvantage in Afghanistan in terms of life expectancy, according to the World Bank (2012), the country has one of the highest maternal mortality rates in the world (460 per 100,000), and more women have reported to be vulnerable and suffering from tuberculosis than men do (WHO 2009a, b). The life expectancy rate at birth for both women and men is improving in the developing world and occurs with demographic change or transition, which is characterised by declines in the rates of mortality and fertility due to advancement in medical treatments and stabilised population growth. However, some argue that while this demographic change is good for women, it may not help to achieve gender equality in other spheres of women's life (McNay 2005).

Another point in the argument is that the life expectancy gap between women and men may now be narrowing both in the developing and developed world. The gender gap in mortality is smaller in developing countries because in many of these countries, women have much lower social status than men (Fuse and Crenshaw 2006). In general, the gender gap is expected to increase in the developing nations due to men benefiting from health advances at all age points. In developed countries, the gender gap is expected to decrease and adversely affects the health of both women and men.

Additionally, UNFPA (2012) informs us that the health gap also narrows or widens based on age and socio-economic status. It can then therefore be argued that the mortality gap varies during different stages of life, and the scale of disparities could increase or decrease. Female- and male-specific problem areas also exist due to gender and cultural norms. For instance, many women die during pregnancy and child birth, one of the crucial stages in a woman's life. It is reported that of the estimated 529,000 maternal deaths each year, 99 % occurs in the developing world. Moreover, it is also reported that just 13 countries are estimated to account for 2/3rds of all these deaths.

The explanation of gender gaps in life expectancy is a complex one, and there is no definitive answer. It is true that women live longer in many parts of the world than men do, but the quality of life which is bounded by gender stereotypes positions women in powerless situations, making women more structurally disadvantaged in relation to access and making use of health services appropriately. As we gather more evidence, it becomes clearer that women and men equally suffer from life-threatening illnesses and diseases caused by social environments and work conditions (Payne and Doyal 2010). Men take the risk with a degree of control; women are more likely to spend more years in poor health or with disability. Social structure is one element that shapes gender mortality and morbidity differences.

Inequalities in Health

Inequalities in health are not only a matter of economic gaps and differences between rich and poor, but it is more complex than that. The need has been stressed to focus on the social basis of health inequalities and sources of the disparities that are diverse (Marmot and Wilkinson 2006). It is important to decipher how social inequalities are produced and maintained strategically. Existing literature and data do not indicate much about the reasons why and how certain social groups are positioned differently and disadvantaged. Information regarding what leads to marginalisation, social exclusion and discrimination and how this relates to health is limited. The detail information of which groups are excluded and why and how do we analyse social exclusion is fragmentary and disconnected to broader theories of power and social positioning.

Social Determinants of Health

Social determinants of health introduced by WHO is one of the leading theoretical frameworks that has gained a lot of attention that sheds some light on the connection around social exclusion, inequalities and health. The social determinants of health model point towards diverse social situations that put certain population groups in vulnerable and marginalised positions. It is noted that addressing social determinants of health allows intersectoral partners to address root causes of ill health. These underlying root causes are 'exclusion, discrimination and inequality'. In other words, healthcare itself is not the only focus, but rather the structural biases that cause health disparities making certain population groups unable to access healthcare. For instance, research from the USA and UK demonstrates the significance of researching race and class inequalities that continue to produce structural

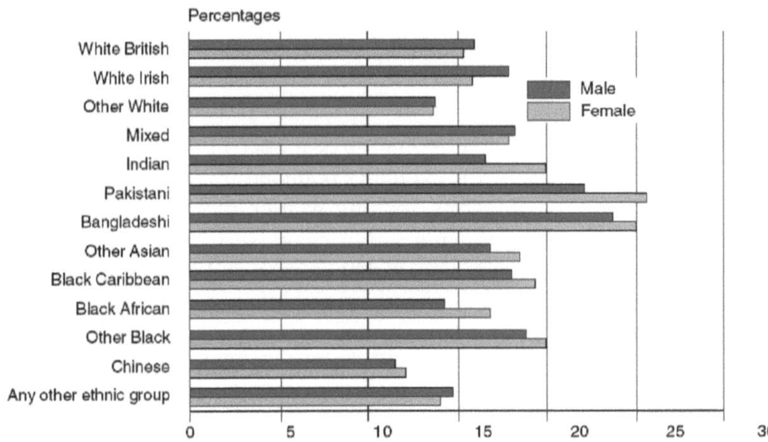

Fig. 11.1 Age-standardised limiting long-term illness: by ethnic group and sex, England and Wales (ONS 2001) discusses in House of Commons Health Committee report (2009)

differences in health in ethnically disadvantaged groups such as Black, Asians, etc. (Nazroo and Williams 2006). Similarly, the UK's Race Equality Foundation clearly states that ethnicity is an important dimension to health inequalities (Fulton 2010). However, there is growing concerns that within the UK, there is lack of empirical information on ethnic inequalities in health. The lack of evidence-based research and initiative to develop race-sensitive data presents limitations and challenges to understanding where exactly inequalities lie and how does that relate to social exclusion. However, what we do know is that certain groups are discriminated against on the basis of their racial and gender identity.

Similarly, the House of Commons Health Committee report (2009) on health inequalities demonstrates disparities in health between ethnic groups. The report showed that Indian, Pakistani and Bangladeshi reported poor health and limiting long-term illness as compared to other groups in England and Wales (See Fig. 11.1). However, the report failed to capture a detailed gender and racial analysis as well as other social categories that could have potentially helped to indicate the causes of inequalities amongst different groups. When ethnic diversity was taken into account, the female and male groups from all mentioned ethnic backgrounds were considered as homogenous categories despite the diverse nature of the UK's population. When gender disparities in health are highlighted in the report, the reference is only made to the illnesses affecting men when clearly it is women across all groups (expect white groups and 'any other ethnic group') who are affected by the negative consequences of health more than men (see Fig. 11.1). There is no acknowledgement let alone discussion of female health issues in the report. It goes to show that the significance of gender inequalities in health is yet to be acknowledged that intersects with race, class, geographical situation and other social categories. Data on gender forms of social advantage in the UK and elsewhere is limited, almost always overshadowed by socio-economic disadvantages such as education and class. Gender has rarely been considered an important variable or aspect to magnify on inequalities in health that affect women just because they are women.

Social Exclusion and Identity

Poverty is one of the major structural factors that position individuals in disadvantaged situations; inequalities can be further exacerbated by other social dimensions. How individuals and population groups are positioned in the society plays a vital role in how health is delivered, accessed and used. Social status, which is relational, and power relations that privileges one group over the other are central. It relates to the identity (assumed, perceived and/or expected) of certain groups of people; identities that are socially produced undermine and devalue certain population groups based on 'who they are (or rather who they are perceived to be)' (Kabeer 2006). As a result of social and economic disparities, certain population groups may have little control and/or power to access and use health services.

Mumtaz et al. (2012) finds social exclusion framework useful to explain disparities in access to maternal health services in Pakistan. They argue that the gendered social structures, processes and relations lead to women being systematically denied resources, and full participation in society become the basis for denial of maternal health services. Social inclusion/exclusion is informed by society and power relations that underlie social meaning, which puts certain groups at increased risk for life-threatening diseases. It is important that we problematise and engage ourselves fully in identity politics when trying to understand changing meanings of gender and theories of social structure that result in producing disparities and inequities in health.

However, it is misleading to consider that women and men to be uniformly disadvantaged in terms of health. Health inequalities should then be understood through the intersecting domains of inclusion, exclusion and identity. The social inclusion/exclusion and identity frameworks allow the exploration of the ways in which social structures interact with one another that fuel marginalisation and vulnerability. These imply explicit and implicit engagement with the theory of difference informed by the feminist theory of intersectionality.

Intersectionality Theory and Decentralization

The social inclusion and exclusion approach provides an uncomplicated way of viewing power relations between two groups. While social determinants of health is a useful model, this acclaimed exposition of inequality fails to capture complexities and diversity of people's lived experiences. Moreover, its knowledge around gender is limited and patchy. In dealing with contemporary inequalities, it is important to look at other concepts and complexities that fail to capture this. The focus should not be on filtering social categories out, but there is a need to deconstruct the social aspects to fully comprehend inequalities. Therefore, it is important to extend beyond this framework to avoid simplistic analysis of gender beings.

Intersectionality Theory

The feminist theory of intersectionality (Crenshaw 1989), which has started to gain some attention in health areas, is central to reconceptualising gender-disadvantaged positions that lends itself to extension beyond economic and biological fitness. In this context, the social categories of gender, race and class itself are not the only feature of justice in health. Other issues such as geography, location, history, disability, sexuality, caste, class and religion influence greater understanding of how inequalities are produced historically and spatially.

Intersectionality theory is concerned with discrimination in circumstances where these inequalities intersect at the same time. This framework has been useful in making social inequalities visible that influence the health status of both women and men. In this theory, one ontological level does not take priority over the other; rather these strands are seen to be intersecting at the same time whereby interconnected inequalities do not operate in isolation.

These inequalities affect one another significantly, for example, you could be a woman, from a certain caste, class and ethnic background; an individual who falls under these categories could be seen in marginalised positions, in which he/she is bound to face inequalities based on individual groups social positioning. In intersectionality, these marginalities intersect at the same time, and one does not take priority over another. The concept is a useful analytical tool in tracing how certain people are positioned as not only different but marginalised. This also means that to understand one position, it is vital to stretch the focus out into other areas with which they intersect. It makes the root causes of inequalities and power imbalances between population groups in health visible. Intersectionality has the ability to create different lived experiences and social realities of people and that intersectionality lets us view endless intersecting social spheres and interests where different divisions of inequality merge and through which these differences can be revealed.

When conducting gender analysis in health, it is important to consider which gender differences (age, sexuality, class, caste, race, location, etc.) will contribute to our understanding of health inequities. It teases out the complex interrelationship between variables or speculating as to their intersections with their social locations. This analysis makes visible the scale and level of inequities and inequalities that exist across different social groupings.

Gender Inclusion in Decentralised Governance

At a very minimum level, decentralization can be defined as transfer of political powers from the central to the local level, which is seen as good governance practice. Lessons learned indicate that delegating responsibility to the local and district levels alone is not working. The process especially in some developing countries is bureaucratic and complex in nature.

It has been argued that a patriarchal system/government managed and run by privileged groups (based on gender, race, class, nationality, sexuality, etc.) undermines the rights of women and socially disadvantaged groups. At the district and local levels, the laws are rooted in the different customs of many different ethnic tribes that make up the district or state (Mahendru 2012). In this context, the laws are enforced according to the cultural demands of each ethno-nationality where many social disadvantaged communities and women feel marginalised and excluded in the political process of decentralised systems.

While devolution of powers is an important gain, many countries are failing to address gender equity and equality appropriately reinforcing social exclusion at governance and programmes levels. A gendered analysis of decentralization reform in Cambodia looks at the issues of representation signposts that women are being excluded in political processes. For instance, in India many women and social disadvantaged groups act as proxy to the privileged (husbands, men and men from higher caste, etc.). The inclusion of women and socially disadvantaged groups is being carried out in a very tokenistic manner. The major impediment to deeper gender equality is the social norms upheld by both women and men within political parties (Sedara et al. 2012).

Case Study 2

An international study on decentralization and gender equality conducted a survey to study the prevalence and inclusion of women in local government from Africa, Latin America and the Caribbean, Asia and developed regions using self-reported country data. The survey showed that the average proportion of women in local councils for the 52 countries reporting was just 15 %. The implication of this data may be that women face greater obstacles to political engagement at the local levels in some contexts because of the intensity of local patriarchal norms.

(Source: UNRISD 2005, Chap. 12)

In this context described above, how do we ensure meaningful participation of the socially excluded groups including women in political process and quest of good governance? How do we incorporate objectives of voice and agency of diverse disadvantaged communities and also highlight the significant challenges that remain barriers to the goals of health and gender equity? How to provide complex understanding of these groups for good governance?

At this juncture what we require is a coherent theoretical framework with human rights-based approach that helps explain the dynamic interrelationships between different groups and pertinent information on the prevalence of women and socially excluded groups as health leaders in government. Intersectionality provides an opportunity to unpack different dimensions of social groups that are spatially and historically bound and power relationships are central to it. An understanding of intersectionality has the capacity to preclude intersectional discrimination and includes gender. It takes individual and group experiences into account. Through intersectionality, greater participation of the socially excluded groups can be understood, and eventually health management can be ensured. It requires information that represents multiple groups and which reflects significant variations within different social groups across genders (Hankivsky et al. 2010). Elsewhere, Hankivsky (2007, p. 159) explicitly suggests that gender should not be privileged over other social axes. This understanding of gender analysis could be seen as presumptuous and inadequate. Therefore, a critical reflection and engagement with social other categories as well as spatial analysis is required. Gender exists in diverse forms in different hierarchical social structures. Engagement with theories of gender and health cannot be disentangled by a tokenistic and 'simplistic' approach.

The main concern in decentralization is implementation of local governance through equity and justice lenses especially those concerning inclusion of social processes to enhance the empowerment of vulnerable and marginalised groups. For instance, gender, caste and tribal remain strong markers of disadvantage in India (Gardener and Subrahmanian 2006). There is deep-rooted discrimination based on social differences of gender, caste and ethnicity. Institutional barriers at local governance level continue to limit inclusion of the disadvantaged groups and women in India. There is a need to highlight social injustices that prevent social inclusion.

Conclusion

This chapter called for the need for greater conceptualisation of and data on gender. It discussed and re-emphasised that poverty alone does not explain inequity in health. It has become increasingly important to use different approaches and engage in theoretical debates outside the traditional ways of looking at health. The first step is to disregard women and men as homogenous categories. Gender in health is multidimensional and intersectional, and the true sense of lived realities of both women and men can be understood by focusing on other social strands and how these different strands interact to produce health inequalities. While certain social groups cannot be considered disadvantaged uniformly, this chapter argued that documenting the experiences of those marginalised and exploring health inequities are important to understand and provide solutions to reaching health equity. There are multiple levels of 'inequalities in health' that are produced due to social positioning of individual and groups. These positionings lead to negative health outcomes such as high rates of maternal mortality. Therefore, relationships between gender and other frameworks such as social exclusion and identity frameworks as well as embodying the use of intersectionality theory for an integrated approach in gender research is required, which has a potential to offer a better situated knowledge of the experiences of marginality. However, there is an increasing recognition that regardless of the progress made to date, significant gaps remain in comprehending fully the root causes of inequities, including the complex ways in which the determinants of health relate, intersect and mutually reinforce one another. The availability of data for analysis is one of the key aspects in order to have a better understanding of which groups are vulnerable and marginalised. Intersectional research and consistently comparable gender disaggregated data should be considered integral to health system strengthening from intersectional and gender perspectives.

Further Discussion and Activity

Question 1: Does decentralising healthcare from intersectional perspectives and social inclusion framework improve health equity and reduces gender inequity?

Question 2: To what extent disaggregated data could be gathered to bring clarity on intersectionality and gender inequity?

Activity

Reflect on a situation where you might have felt different or excluded due to who you are (age, class, gender, race) and where you were (public space, private space, work settings, school, university, hospital).

Hint: You might have felt different because you could not relate to a group, situation and/or a place.

Recommended Reading

Doyal, L. (2001). Sex, gender, and health: The need for a new approach. *British Medical Journal, 323*, 1061–1063.

Readers may find "Sex and health: the biology of risk" section of this paper useful and interesting.

Hankivsky, O., Reid, C., Cormier, R., Varcoe, C., Clark, N., Benoit, C, et al. (2010). Exploring the promises of intersectionality for advancing women's health research. *International Journal for Equity in Health, 9*(1), 5.

Hankivsky et al. *paper on intersectionality in the context Canadian women's health investigates practical challenges involved in applying an intersectionality paradigm to health research.*

Kabeer, N. (2006). Poverty, social exclusion and the MDGs: The challenges of "durable inequalities" in the Asian context. *IDS Bulletin 2006, 37*, 64–78

With focus on marginalised and vulnerable communities, Kabeer presents perspectives from Asia on social exclusion and identity frameworks. She explains exclusion and the quality of health care provision often biased against poor and marginalised groups with its relevance to gender

Marmot, M., & Wilkinson, R. G. (2006). *The social determinants of health* (2nd ed.) Oxford: Oxford University Press.

This book discusses number of determinants of health and discusses inequalities in health at a great health. Though its understanding of gender is limited, readers may find it a useful source.

Acknowledgement I would like to thank Professor Janet Holland London South Bank University (UK) for her valuable input and taking time to look at this chapter.

References

Annandale, E., & Hunt, K. (2000). *Gender inequalities in health: Research at the crossroads*. Buckingham: Open University Press.

Crenshaw, K. (1989) *Demarginalizing the intersection of race and sex: A black feminist critique of antidiscrimination doctrine, feminist theory and antiracist politics*. University of Chicago Legal Forum 138–67.

Connell, R. (2012). Gender, health and theory: Conceptualizing the issue, in local and world perspective. *Social Science and Medicine, 74*(11), 1675. 1683.

Fulton, R. (2010). *A race equality foundation briefing paper: Ethnic monitoring: Is health equality possible without it?* London: Race Equality Foundation.

Fuse, K., & Crenshaw, E. M. (2006). Gender imbalance in infant mortality: A cross-national study of social structure and female infanticide. *Social Science and Medicine, 62*(2), 360–374.

Gardener, J., & Subrahmanian, R. (2006). *Tackling social exclusion in health and education: Case studies from Asia/Summary Report*. London: DFID.

GRAVIS. (2010). *Women miners in Rajasthan, India: A reflection on their life, challenges and future*. Rajasthan: GRAVIS.

Hankivsky, O. (2007). Gender based analysis and health policy: The need to rethink outdated strategies. In M. Morrow, O. Hankivsky, & C. Varcoe (Eds.), *Women's health in Canada: Critical theory, policy and practice* (pp. 143–168). Toronto, ON: University of Toronto Press.

Hankivsky, O., Reid, C., Cormier, R., Varcoe, C., Clark, N., Benoit, C., et al. (2010). Exploring the promises of intersectionality for advancing women's health research. *International Journal for Equity in Health, 9*(1), 5.

Holland, J., Ramazanoglu, C., Sharpe, S., & Thomson, R. (1998). *Male in the head*. London: The Tufnell Press.

House of Commons Health Committee report. (2009). *Health inequalities: Third report of session 2008–09*. London: The Stationery Office Limited.

Kabeer, N. (2006). Poverty, social exclusion and the MDGs: the challenges of "durable inequalities" in the Asian context. *IDS Bull, 2006*(37), 64–78.

Kolip, P. (2010). Primary prevention and health promotion: Towards gender sensitive interventions. In E. Kuhlmann & E. Annandale (Eds.), *The Palgrave handbook of gender and healthcare* (pp. 337–354). Basingstoke: Palgrave.

Kuhlmann, E., & Annandale, E. (2010). *The Palgrave handbook of gender and healthcare*. Basingstoke: Palgrave.

Mahendru, R. (2012). *Population trends and policy options in selected developing countries (Sub-Saharan Africa and Asia)*. Bangladesh: Partners in Population Development.

Marmot, M., & Wilkinson, R. G. (2006). *The social determinants of health* (2nd ed.). Oxford: Oxford University Press.
McNay, K. (2005). The implications of the demographic transition for women, girls and gender equality: a review of developing country evidence. *Progress in Development Studies, 5*(2), 115.
Mumtaz, Z., Salway, S., Shanner, L., Zaman, S., & Laing, L. (2012). Addressing disparities in maternal health care in Pakistan: gender, class and exclusion. *BMC Pregnancy and Childbirth, 12*, 80.
Nazroo, J. Y., & Williams, D. R. (2006). The social determination of ethnic/racial inequalities in health. In M. Marmot & R. G. Wilkinson (Eds.), *The social determinants of health* (2nd ed., pp. 238–266). Oxford: Oxford University Press.
Obot, I. S., & Room, R. (2005). *Alcohol, gender and drinking problems: Perspectives from low and middle income countries*. Geneva, Switzerland: World Health organisation, Department of Mental Health and Substance Abuse.
ONS (2001) Age-standardised limiting long-term illness: By ethnic group and sex, England and Wales. Official national Statistics [online] Available at: http://www.ons.gov.uk/ons/CCI/nugget.asp?ID=1007&Pos=6&ColRank=2&Rank=1000
Payne, S., & Doyal, L. (2010). Re-visiting gender justice in health and health care. In E. Kuhlmann & E. Annandale (Eds.), *The Palgrave handbook of gender and healthcare* (pp. 21–35). Basingstoke: Palgrave.
Peden, M., Scurfield, R., Sleet, D., Mohan, D., Hyder, A., Jarawan, E., & Mathers, C. (2004). *World report on road traffic injury prevention*. Geneva: World Health Organisation.
Sedara, K., Ojendal, J., Nareth, C., & Tem, L. Y. (2012). *A gendered analysis of decentralisation reform in Cambodia*. Cambodia: CDRI.
UNFPA. (2012). *Changing levels and trends in mortality: The role of patterns of death by cause*. New York: UNFPA.
UNRISD. (2005). *Decentralization and gender equality, in gender equality striving for justice in an unequal world*. New York: UNRISD/UN Publications.
WHO. (2004). *Global status report on alcohol*. Geneva: World Health Organization.
WHO (2008a) Global burden of disease: 2004 Update (online) World Health Organisation. Available at: http://www.who.int/healthinfo/global_burden_disease/GBD_report_2004update_full.pdf (Accessed 14 May 2013)
WHO (2008b) Equity in access to public health [online] World Health Organisation. Available at: http://209.61.208.233/en/Section1430/Section1439/Section1638/Section1746/Section2442_13725.htm (Accessed 15 May 2013)
WHO. (2009a). *WHO Report 2009. Global tuberculosis control: Epidemiology, strategy, financing*. Geneva: World Health Organization.
WHO. (2009b). *Women's health: Fact sheet Number 334*. Available at: http://www.who.int/mediacentre/factsheets/fs334/en/ [Accessed 14 May 2013]
World Bank. (2012). Maternal mortality ratio (modeled estimate, per 100,000 live births) [online] Available at: http://data.worldbank.org/indicator/SH.STA.MMRT Last Accessed [15 May 2013]
WorldBank. (2011). *Life expectancy at birth, total (years)* [online] Available at: http://data.worldbank.org/indicator/SP.DYN.LE00.IN [Accessed 14 May 2013]
Yin, S. (2007). *Gender disparities in health and mortality* [online] Population Reference Bureau. Available at: http://www.prb.org/Articles/2007/genderdisparities.aspx [Accessed 14 May 2013]

Chapter 12
Decentralization of Health Systems: Challenges and Global Issues of the Twenty-First Century

Thomas J. Bossert

Abstract Decentralization of health systems is a growing trend in most nations. However, there are a series of new challenges that face these processes of decentralization. To assess these challenges, this chapter first starts with a definition of decentralization that defines *who* gets more choice (deconcentration or devolution) and *how much* choice they get over *what functions,* which we call "decision space." It is also important to assess the *capacities* of those who receive more choice and the *accountability* they have toward the national authorities and the local population of beneficiaries. The major new challenges to the processes of decentralization reviewed in this chapter are national health insurance and universal coverage, growth of the private sector, epidemiological and demographic changes, and new structures of governance and accountability. It concludes with policy recommendations which suggest the need to balance "decision space" for local authorities with realistic development of their capacities, reserving some key functions to the national authorities. It is also important to push forward a research agenda to assess the best mix of the elements of decentralization that are most likely to achieve better health system performance.

After Reading This Chapter You Will Be Able to

- *Use the concepts of deconcentration, devolution, "decision space," capacities, and accountability to analyze characteristics of decentralized health systems.*
- *Understand the challenges that universal health coverage, growth of the private sector, epidemiological and demographic change, and new forms of governance have for the process of decentralization.*

T.J. Bossert (✉)
Department of Global Health and Population, Harvard School of Public Health,
665 Huntington Avenue, Building I, Room 1207, Boston, MA, USA
e-mail: tbossert@hsph.harvard.edu

K. Regmi (ed.), *Decentralizing Health Services: A Global Perspective*,
DOI 10.1007/978-1-4614-9071-5_12,

- *Recommend a balanced approach to decentralization which specifies some functions to be centralized while others may be decentralized.*

Introduction

There is no doubt that the trend of national health system change in the future is toward greater decentralization. Almost every country's national strategic plan for health involves at least some commitment to decentralization. While there may be some specific cases of greater centralization, or recentralization, processes driven both within and outside the sector are pushing toward more local decision making about the health sector. Recent significant decentralization has occurred in Pakistan which after several earlier attempts has significantly reduced central control over the health system, even for a period of time eliminating the federal ministry of health and granting most functions to the provinces (WHO et al. 2012). India has charged its already partly decentralized states with decentralizing further to districts and blocks. Latin American countries, including Chile, Colombia, Mexico, and Brazil, have been leaders in the process of decentralization. And in Africa, Nigeria and Ghana have historically been in the forefront of decentralization. South Africa is currently considering a similar shift toward more local control.

Analysis of Decentralization

Decentralization is above all about shifting the choices of policy and implementation from central authorities to subnational governmental levels. The classic approach, first published by Rondinelli and adopted by Mills in a monograph for WHO, offers a typology of:

- "Deconcentration," which shifts choice to lower administrative levels of a national institution such as districts within the ministry of health
- "Devolution," which shifts choice to lower levels of government like state or municipal governments
- "Delegation," which shifts choice to semiautonomous organizations like boards of health
  (Rondinelli 1981; Mills et al. 1990)

This typology tells *who* gets more choice.

I have added to this analysis the concept of "decision space" which views decentralization as shifting a degree of choice (narrow, moderate, or wide) for a series of functions (financing, service delivery, human resources, access rules, and governance) to the subnational levels (Bossert 1998). This answers the question of *how much* choice over *what* functions.

In addition to these ways of analyzing decentralization, two other concepts are important for decentralization to be effective in improving health system performance: *capacity* and *accountability* (Bossert and Mitchell 2011). Both the central authorities and the subnational administrative institutions need to have the requisite capacities to make good decisions within the "decision space" they are allowed. For instance, if decision space is increased in financing and in human resources, management capacity in these areas is needed at the level that receives additional decision-making choice. This does not necessarily mean that greater decision space need to wait until capacity is developed—often it is necessary to have more choice to develop those capacities. At the same time, those who are granted more choice need to be accountable for better performance by both the local beneficiary population and the national authorities. New mechanisms of accountability such as pay for performance, or management contracting for accountability to higher authorities, or local governments or community participation boards with ability to sanction health officials for failure to perform as required need to be developed and implemented (Mitchell and Bossert 2010).

New Challenges

There have been recent waves of changes in health systems which pose challenges to the overall trend toward greater decentralization. Here we examine the processes of:

- The introduction of new social insurance systems under the current banner of *universal coverage.*
- The growth of private sector, both for provision of services and for insurance, is also a major challenge for the decentralization of public administration in health.
- New structures for governance, especially at the facility level, also pose a challenge.
- Ultimately the epidemiological and demographic shifts toward NCDs and aging population also may require changes in decentralization.

National Health Insurance

The current wave of interest in universal coverage and national health insurance (NHI) raises new problems for decentralization (World Health Organization 2010; Kutzin 2013). NHI might be implemented either by a decentralized health insurance agency or utilize state or district level authorities as a "wholesaler" which contract with the insurance agency and then organize the providers in their geographic area. However, many countries are adopting an insurance system in which the insurer is a sole payer which contracts directly with the provider facilities or individual health professionals, bypassing the local offices of the ministries of health or the local governments. While some functions such as general public health, promotion, and information systems may remain in a decentralized public system, this shift to insurance as direct payer reduces the role of the decentralized public entities.

Growth of the Private Sector

Similarly as health systems that were previously dominated by the public provider services move to a more mixed system with a greater role for the private sector, the public entities in a decentralized system may shift toward a more regulatory role than one of direct provision or, at least, reorient to manage a public/private partnership (see Reich 2002). In this case, developing the capacities of local government administrations in the complex issues of contracting with the private sector will become more important than they were when local administrations only managed public facilities.

Epidemiological and Demographic Changes

Demographic and epidemiological changes such as the aging of the population and the growth of noncommunicable diseases (NCDs) abetted by obesity (leading in many countries the "double burden of disease") will also affect the processes of decentralization. This poses a challenge to many systems that developed primary care to address mainly communicable diseases and maternal and child health and devolved primary care to the municipal level. Now there is a growing need to revamp primary care to introduce more prevention and promotion specifically for NCDs and rehabilitation and maintenance of chronic disease treatments at the primary care level. The challenge will be to introduce new types of primary care services throughout a decentralized system.

Governance Issues and Accountability

Governance issues are becoming more complex with the choices that centralized governments may have to make as they decentralize. The first choice, as Rondinelli posed, is the choice of whether to decentralize to local governments (devolution) or only to "deconcentrate" by granting greater choice to local administrative units of the ministry of health. In addition, as countries grant more "autonomy" to their public hospitals, the issue of governing boards for those facilities becomes important. Just creating a board may not be enough to assure accountability and better management; the composition and the specific responsibilities need to be carefully chosen in order to improve the performance of those facilities (Bossert 2008). It is also important to revisit the mechanisms that have traditionally been recommended to improve accountability of local administrations to their beneficiaries. It is not obvious that local elected officials will respond to the demand and needs of the broad population or especially to the most vulnerable. The characteristics of the local government vary considerably, and a focus on improving those characteristics may be necessary. Community participation committees also may not be effectively designed to enhance accountability as they often have been controlled by the local health staff to provide voluntary labor more than for social auditing. The role of social capital in communities may be important to evaluate and strengthen in order to improve accountability at the local level (Brune and Bossert 2009). And finally, addressing the issue of corruption is essential to improving the legitimacy and the effectiveness of local administration of health systems (Bossert and Mitchell 2011; Lewis 2006).

Capacity Development

Each of these challenges above raises capacity issues (Bossert and Mitchell 2011). NHI and private sector growth raise the need to develop the payer or contractor roles with the separation of financing from provision and also the possibility in many systems of contracting with private sector providers. The epidemiological and demographic shift will require new technical tasks as well as more social engagement to develop promotion programs for NCDs. In addition to these new challenges, there continues to be a need to deal with the traditional administrative strengthening in both technical and management areas that for many countries have been found lacking.

Policy and Research Needs

If I am right about the trend toward decentralization and the new challenges posed by NHI, private sector growth, and epidemiological and demographic changes, then it will be important to define more clearly the functions that should be retained at the center and those that will improve health system performance if they are decentralized to local officials. It will also be important to define the governance structures at local level that are most appropriate.

The evidence about the effectiveness of decentralization in general is and has been mixed. Many case studies have shown both the advantages and disadvantages of decentralization (Prud'Homme 1995; Faguet 2012). Much of the literature on decentralization exposes the biases of the authors rather than providing carefully evaluated studies of the actual impacts of the decentralization itself. It is notoriously difficult to demonstrate the effect of decentralization on goals and objectives we might have for policies. Many factors affect these goals and objectives, and it is difficult to isolate the effect of decentralization. Few countries are willing to introduce decentralization through methods similar to random trials that might provide some clearer evidence of causality.

While there is a current ongoing systematic review of the literature on decentralization, using methods of the Cochrane collection, its results are not yet completed. One of the most interesting recent studies of decentralization in general by JP Faguet concludes that the trend of the literature is more in favor of decentralization while recognizing many problems with the process (Faguet 2012). The Faguet study of Bolivia shows that the importance of the characteristics of local government—in particular, those that reduce elite capture and increase democratic responsiveness—is the major factor in the effectiveness of decentralization. This finding echoes earlier findings of Robert Putnam in his much earlier study of decentralization in Italy (Putnam 1993). My own work on decentralization in the health sector suggests that there are some functions that should be retained at the central level and others that might be decentralized but only if certain conditions can be created (Bossert et al. 2007). This is not an argument that we need to wait until local governments have those conditions, but we need to think about how to pace the process of decentralization so that there are incentives for the creation of capacities and conditions, as well as the support necessary for increasing those capacities and providing the conditions. While it would be useful to have more clear empirical evidence of the right way to do decentralization, I will offer here some tentative suggestions about the future processes.

First it is important to **clarify the goals of decentralization policy** in terms of improved health system performance. This sector perspective is in contrast to those who seek decentralization because they want greater power in the hands of local populations—in other words, those who seek decentralization as a goal in itself rather than a means toward the end of better health system performance. Roberts et al. (2003) offer a clear set of objectives for health system performance that might be useful.

Second, there are **some functions that generally will be better performed if they are retained, or restored, to the central authorities**:

- Perhaps the most important is to **have uniform information systems** (on epidemiology, utilization, financing, and management) to provide consistent and comparable information for both local and central authorities. Without strong, valid, and comparative information, both effective management at the local levels and clear accountability to the central level for performance assessment will be severely hampered.
- Along with the routine information systems, there needs to also put in place **strong auditing of financing** in order to reduce opportunities for corruption.
- Since both clinical protocols and quality assurance processes require significant and up-to-date knowledge and information, there should be **a strong central hand in defining the norms and standards for quality** in clinical and prevention programs.
- Some **basic financial allocations decisions** should also be made at the central level in order to assure greater equity in territorial distribution and to protect the funding for priority programs, particularly those devoted to prevention and promotion.

- Finally, to reduce patronage and nepotism, strong centrally defined processes of recruitment, promotion, and termination should be developed into **a merit-oriented human resource management process that has internal and external checks and transparency**.

Third, **functions that can be decentralized**, if there is reasonable expectation that the central functions will be developed, include:

- A **range of flexibility in implementing budgets and plans** according to local conditions
- **Opportunities for managers to provide incentives to motivate the workforce**
- **Some service delivery decisions** such as bed assignments, timing of services and campaigns, and location of facilities
- **Introduction of programs to address local priority health problems**

Case Example: Pakistan: Too Much Decentralization?

Through a constitutional amendment, a very radical process of devolution to the provinces was initiated in Pakistan in 2010. Prior to the amendment, there had been a "concurrent list" of functions shared by the provinces and the federal government; however, the federal government exercised most of those functions leaving little actual "decision space" for the provinces. The amendment radically reduced the list of functions that the federal government could exercise, leaving most functions in the hands of the provinces. In implementing the amendment, the government first eliminated the federal ministry of health and distributed the few remaining federal responsibilities among several general ministries. This caused tremendous difficulties for both the national health policies and for the provinces, especially in areas where coordination was needed. In response to this negative experience, the ministry of health was restored in 2013, and a more appropriate balance of responsibilities between the federal and provincial authorities established (WHO et al. 2012).

Conclusion

The complexity of decentralization has traditionally left policy makers with difficult choices related to decision space, capacities, and accountability. The new challenges of this century (universal coverage and national health insurance, growth of the private sector, epidemiological and demographic changes, and the challenge of new governance and accountability mechanisms) will only make these decisions more complicated. The secular trend toward decentralization will require careful consideration of these choices and not quick fix solutions.

Discussion Questions

1. Consider a country you know well. What is the current "decision space" for a subnational administrative level (e.g., state, province, municipality)? How would you change that "decision space" in the face of a new national health insurance policy, growth of the private sector, and/or epidemiological and demographic changes?
2. If you make those changes, what new efforts in capacity building and development of new governance and accountability structures would you recommend?

Recommended Reading

1. Faguet, J-P. (2012). *Decentralization and popular democracy: Governance from below in Bolivia*. Ann Arbor: University of Michigan Press—the most recent overview of the general literature on decentralization and an excellent case study of decentralization in Bolivia.
2. Bossert, T. (1998, November). Analyzing the decentralization of health systems in developing countries: decision space, innovation and performance. *Social Science and Medicine*—a now classic article introducing the concept of "decision space" and application to the health system in Colombia.
3. Mitchell, A., & Bossert, T. (2010). Decentralization, governance and health system performance: "Where you stand depends on where you sit". *Development Policy Review 28*(6), 669–691—a recent review of literature and cases on governance in health system decentralization.

References

Bossert, T. (1998). Analyzing the decentralization of health systems in developing countries: Decision space, innovation and performance. *Social Science and Medicine, 47*(10), 1513–1527.

Bossert, T. (2008) *Decentralization and governance in health*. Bethesda: Health Systems 20/20 Project, June 2008.

Bossert, T., Bowser, D., & Amenyah, J. (2007). Is decentralization good for logistics systems? Evidence on essential medicine logistics from Ghana and Guatemala. *Health Policy and Planning, 22*(2), 73–82.

Bossert, T., & Mitchell, A. (2011). Health sector decentralization and local decision-making: Decision space, institutional capacities and accountability in Pakistan. *Social Science and Medicine, 72*(1), 39–48.

Brune, N., & Bossert, T. (2009). Building social capital in post-conflict communities: Evidence from Nicaragua. *Social Science and Medicine, 68*(5), 885–893.

Faguet, J.-P. (2012). *Decentralization and popular democracy: Governance from below in Bolivia*. Ann Arbor: University of Michigan Press.

Kutzin, J. (2013) Health financing for universal coverage and health system performance: Concepts and implications for policy. *Bulletin of the World Health Organization*. Available at: http://www.who.int/bulletin/online_first/12-113985.pdf (Accessed on 7/7/2013).

Lewis, M. (2006). *Governance and corruption in public health systems*. Washington, DC: Center for Global Development Working Paper.

Mills, A., et al. (1990). *Health system decentralization: Concepts, issues and country experience*. Geneva: World Health Organization.

Mitchell, A., & Bossert, T. (2010). Decentralization, governance and health system performance: Where you stand depends on where you sit. *Development Policy Review, 28*(6), 669–691.

Prud'Homme, R. (1995). On the dangers of decentralization. *World Bank Research Observer, 10*, 210–216.

Putnam, R. (1993). *Making democracy work*. Princeton: Princeton University Press.

Reich, M. R. (2002). *Public–private partnerships for public health*. Cambridge: Harvard Center for Population and Development Studies, distributed by Harvard University Press.

Roberts, M., Hsiao, W., Reich, M., & Berman, P. (2003). *Getting health reform right*. Oxford: Oxford University Press.

Rondinelli, D. A. (1981). Government decentralization in comparative perspective: Theory and practice in developing countries. *International Review of Administrative Sciences, 47*, 133–145.

World Health Organization. (2010). *The world health report—Health systems financing: the path to universal coverage*. Geneva: World Health Organization.

World Health Organization, World Bank, DFID, USAID-TAUH, Joint Mission. (2012). *Devolution of the Health Sector following the 18th Amendment to the Constitution of Pakistan: Opportunities and Challenges*. Geneva: World Health Organization.

Index

K. Regmi (ed.), *Decentralizing Health Services: A Global Perspective*,
DOI 10.1007/978-1-4614-9071-5, © Springer Science+Business Media New York 2014

MIX
Papier aus verantwortungsvollen Quellen
Paper from responsible sources
FSC® C105338

If you have any concerns about our products,
you can contact us on
ProductSafety@springernature.com

In case Publisher is established outside the EU,
the EU authorized representative is:
Springer Nature Customer Service Center GmbH
Europaplatz 3, 69115 Heidelberg, Germany

Printed by Libri Plureos GmbH
in Hamburg, Germany